MW01114366

BALANCED SCORECARD IN THE FEDERAL GOVERNMENT

BALANCED SCORECARD IN THE FEDERAL GOVERNMENT

James B. Whittaker

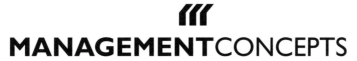

MANAGEMENTCONCEPTS

Vienna, Virginia

Management Concepts, Inc.
8230 Leesburg Pike, Suite 800
Vienna, Virginia 22182
Phone: (703) 790-9595
Fax: (703) 790-1371
Web: www.managementconcepts.com

Printed in the United States of America

Library of Congress Cataloging-in-Publication Data

Whittaker, James B.
  Balanced scorecard in the federal government / James B. Whittaker.
    p. cm.
  Includes index.
  ISBN 1-56726-097-7 (hc.)
  1. Administrative agencies—United States—Management—Evaluation.
2. Administrative agencies—United States—Planning—Evaluation.   3. Government productivity—United States—Evaluation.   4. United States. Government Performance and Results Act of 1993.   I. Title.

JK421.W453   2000
352.4'39'0973—dc21

00-063815

About the Author

James B. Whittaker is a well-known author and lecturer about the Government Performance and Results Act of 1993 (GPRA). His commitment to strategic planning, performance measurement, and leadership in the federal government spans more than 40 years. He has held executive positions in the public sector and currently holds executive positions in the private sector. He retired from the U.S. Navy with the rank of Rear Admiral. He was responsible for developing and implementing strategic plans and performance plans for a variety of organizations, and he has defended these plans before the U.S. Congress. He has used the theories in a practical manner to deal with a variety of oversight agencies, including the Office of Management and Budget, the General Accounting Office, and the General Services Administration. As program manager for four of the largest and most successful automatic data processing projects in the federal government, he was responsible for awarding contracts of more than $4 billion. He was also responsible for the reengineering of three major business processes that procured, stored, and issued an inventory valued at more than $50 billion. He was appointed Acting Deputy Assistant Secretary of Defense for Systems under President Reagan.

Dr. Whittaker is currently a founder and officer in several high-technology companies and a consultant to the General Accounting Office and the Office of Personnel Management. He has been the primary lecturer on strategic planning in the Office of Personnel Management Senior Executive Service development program for more than 10 years and the primary GPRA lecturer since the law was passed. In 1994, he gave several Government Performance and Results Act pilot courses to support the General Accounting Office, the Office of Management and Budget, and the Office of Personnel Management. He is currently engaged in developing and implementing several strategic plans and performance plans in the civil agencies and the Department of Defense. In the past several years, clients have included the Board of Governors of the Federal Reserve System, the United Nations Development Program, the U.S. Department of Agriculture, the Centers for Disease Control, the National Institutes of Health, the World Bank, Defense Supply Center, Columbus, Ohio, Defense Reutilization and Marketing Service, Battle Creek, Michigan, the Census Department, the U.S. Department of Education, the U.S. Department of the Treasury, the Defense Mapping Agency, the Department of the Army, and the Immigration and Naturalization Service.

He has a Ph.D. and an M.B.A. (with distinction) from the University of Michigan and a B.S. from the University of Kansas. He is the author of *Strategic Planning in the Federal Government: GPRA Best Practices, Strategic Planning in a Rapidly Changing Environment, Strategic Planning in the U.S. Government, The Government Performance and Results Act of 1993, and The Government Performance and Results Act, Second Edition.* Dr. Whittaker has developed and taught several management seminars on the faculty of the Management Education Department of the Graduate School of Business Administration of The University of Michigan. He has also been an adjunct member of the faculty of The George Washington University, the Catholic University of America, and Georgetown University, among others.

Table of Contents

Preface ix

Chapter 1. Overview 1
Time for the Balanced Scorecard 2
The Balanced Scorecard for the Federal Government 2
Why This Time May Be Different 3

Chapter 2. The Balanced Scorecard in the Private Sector:
Measuring Business Strategy 5
Financial Perspective 5
Customer Perspective 6
Internal Business Perspective 7
Learning and Growth Perspective 8
Conclusion 10

Chapter 3. The Balanced Scorecard at the Federal Aviation
Administration Logistics Center 11
FAALC Strategic Plan for 1994 11
FAALC Strategic Plan for 1997 16
FAALC Strategic Plan for 1999–2002 26

Chapter 4. The Balanced Scorecard at the Naval Undersea
Warfare Center 41
Naval Undersea Warfare Center 1998 Strategic Plan 41
NUSC Strategic Management Process 51
NUWC Newport Division 1998 Strategic Plan 53
NUWC Newport Division 1998 Strategic Plan Brochure 69
NUWC Newport Division 5-Year Planning Proccess 72
Newspaper Article: Five-Year Planning Explained in One Easy Lesson 75

Chapter 5. The Balanced Scorecard at the Veterans Benefits
Administration 79
Systematic Technical Accuracy Review Program for Compensation and
Pension Claims Processing 79

Chapter 6. Balanced Measures at the Internal Revenue Service 87
Commissioner's Testimony 87
The IRS Balanced Measurement System 90
Organizational Performance Management and the IRS Balanced
Measurement System 107

Chapter 7. Systems Executive Officer for Manpower and Personnel:
Strategic Direction and Performance Measurement 115

Chapter 8. A Report on Managing Performance in the Government **127**
  Interagency Work Group on Performance Management 127

Chapter 9. Best Practices in Performance Measurement **143**
  Balancing Measures: Best Practices in Performance Management 143

**Chapter 10. The Balanced Scorecard in Information Technology
  at the General Services Administration** **153**
  Eight Steps to Develop and Use Information Technology Performance
    Measures Effectively 153

**Chapter 11. The Balanced Scorecard in Information Technology
  at the General Accounting Office** **161**
  Measuring Performance and Demonstrating Results of Information
    Technology Investments 161

**Chapter 12. The Balanced Scorecard in Procurement—
  Two Case Examples** **175**
  PEA Guide to the Balanced Scorecard 175
  Department of Transportation's Procurement Balanced Scorecard 191

**Chapter 13. The Balanced Scorecard at the National Oceanic
  and Atmospheric Administration** **205**
  Systems Corporate Balanced Scorecard 205
  Acquisitions Corporate Balanced Scorecard 207
  Human Resources Corporate Balanced Scorecard 209

**Chapter 14. The Balanced Scorecard in Human Resources
  at the Department of Energy** **213**
  Strategic Measurement System for DOE Contractor Human
    Resources (SMS[HR]): A Comprehensive Approach to Tailored Strategic
    HR Planning 213

Chapter 15. Key Practices Driving Balanced Scorecard Outcomes **223**
  Balanced Scorecard in Government 2000: Key Practices Driving Balanced
    Scorecard Outcomes 223

**Chapter 16. The Future of the Balanced Scorecard in the Federal
  Government** **231**

**Appendix A: Federal Aviation Administration Logistics Center,
  Oklahoma City** **233**

**Appendix B: Veterans Benefits Administration Systematic
  Technical Accuracy Review (STAR) Checklist—Rating** **239**

**Appendix C: Attachments on the Department of Transportation's
  Balanced Scorecard** **253**

Appendix D: Balanced Scorecard for a Contractor **267**

Index **275**

Preface

This book is the second in a new series about the Government Performance and Results Act of 1993 (GPRA), which President Clinton signed into law in August 1993. GPRA requires a dramatic difference in federal government operations to achieve full compliance.

Since 1993, federal organizations have been approaching the implementation of GPRA in a variety of ways. Starting in 1994, several hundred GPRA pilot projects were undertaken as various federal organizations prepared for the first full year of implementation in their own way. This series of books will document how well the federal government is doing in implementing GPRA. The first book established a baseline for strategic planning in the federal government. This second book describes and documents the results of implementation.

The federal government is making progress in using new concepts to implement GPRA. Some organizations and individual functions are using Kaplan and Norton's Balanced Scorecard, modified for the federal government. Other organizations and individual functions are developing a concept called "Balanced Measures." The strength of these new efforts is that they focus on more than just "bottom-line" financial results. It is difficult to focus solely on bottom-line financial results when a vast majority of federal organizations do not operate in a "profit" environment. It therefore makes sense for the federal government to broaden the Balanced Scorecard approach that Kaplan and Norton have used in their pacesetting private sector work.

This book addresses two major topics. The first responds to questions such as: How are the Balanced Scorecard and Balanced Measures being implemented at the organizational level? How long have activities been using these concepts? How have they applied them across the organization? Just as important is the next area, which responds to questions such as: How have functions within the total organization applied these concepts? How have they been applied in the human resources function? How have they been applied in the procurement function? A variety of original case material included in each of the chapters shows how Balanced Scorecards and Balanced Measures have been used over the past several years.

These "real-world" documents offer insights and ideas about what you should do in your particular federal government situation. Finding good ideas in other parts of the federal government or the private sector and adapting them to use in federal government organizations should not be a source of concern. Attempts to "reinvent the wheel" should be minimized in these times of scarce resources, particularly when good ideas are readily available.

This series of books is intended to provide organizations a wealth of data and information on how to improve the performance of the federal government. The books provide personal insight on experiences encountered and identify Web sites containing more detail on the particular organization or function covered.

Special thanks go to John Hirsch, the primary author of Chapter 14, and Sharon Caudle, the author of Chapter 15. Their sharing of this critical material with the federal workforce is most appreciated. Thanks also go to Kristen Noyes for her outstanding research support and to Doug Miller for his excellent production support.

Any inaccuracies or omissions are mine alone. For suggested improvements to future editions or for any detailed questions you have about this book or this series, please contact me through the Internet at JamesBW238@AOL.com or call/fax me at 703-416-8616.

James B. Whittaker
October 2000
Arlington, Virginia

CHAPTER 1
Overview

The U.S. federal government is in the midst of a massive change in the way it does business. For decades, the primary federal government driver has been the budget. Unfortunately, this may never change. However, in August 1993 Congress passed legislation, signed into law by President Clinton, entitled the Government Performance and Results Act of 1993 (GPRA).

This law, which the federal government has been implementing for the past 7 years, sets the stage for the federal government to be managed and measured in different ways. First, it mandates new documents. Rather than being driven by the budget, the law requires agencies of the federal government to have long-range strategic plans. These plans must encompass at least 5 years plus the budget year, or a total minimum of 6 years. The strategic plans are to be driven by the mission of the agency and developed and implemented in consultation with Congress, stakeholders, customers, and employees of the organizations.

Next, the long-range strategic plans, which might span 15 or even 20 years in duration, are to drive the budget. This is a critical change. Anyone who has been a part of government for even a few months knows how important it is to spend funds allocated to an organization in order to get more funds next year. Clearly, federal government incentives in the past have been flawed. GPRA has the potential to correct these problems.

The primary aims of GPRA are to ensure that strategic planning drives budgeting and that resource decisions reflect strategic priorities, not just any "fire storm" that occurs. Agencies must establish long-term priorities and then accomplish them.

Next, the law sets forth a requirement for another new document—a performance plan—to guide the transition from the strategic plan with its long-term goals that are updated at least every 3 years, to what needs to be accomplished over the short term—specifically, in the next fiscal year. The performance plan, which is developed for each fiscal year, sets forth the annual goals and objectives that are derived from the long-term strategic plan. It is this annual performance plan that drives the budget of the government organization.

Six months after the end of each fiscal year, government agencies must report on how well they did in accomplishing annual goals and objectives. This report is due each year on the March 31st following the end of the fiscal year. Fiscal Year (FY) 1999, which ended in September 1999, was the first execution year of GPRA across the federal government. On March 31, 2000, performance reports were submitted on performance against the 1999 annual performance plans.

The transition from the old way of doing things to the new, results-oriented planning atmosphere has been varied. In the summer of 1997, the General Accounting Office (GAO) predicted that "the results of the GPRA Implementation will be uneven."[1] GAO was right.

---

[1]General Accounting Office. *The Government Performance and Results Act: 1997 Implementation Will Be Uneven.* Washington, D.C.: GAO, 1997. Report GGD-97-109.

The level of senior management attention, management involvement, and seriousness, as well as the effectiveness of the implementation, varied widely across the federal government. This finding was true not only on the first set of strategic plans analyzed by GAO and graded by Congress, but also on the performance plans. However, progress was achieved across the board.

TIME FOR THE BALANCED SCORECARD

GPRA established the potential for major change in the way of doing business in most parts of the federal government, most certainly in the executive and legislative branches. The GPRA requirements have been executed with varying levels of results.

While the federal government has been undergoing a major learning effort to "turn around the ship" and have the budget driven by the organization's mission and long-term goals, change has also been occurring in the private sector. Starting about 10 years ago, there was concern that private sector organizations did not have the appropriate balance in their strategies and management systems. First, there was too much emphasis on the short term rather than the long term. Second, there was too much emphasis on financial measures rather than non-financial measures. Third, more emphasis was needed on leading indicators rather than lagging indicators. Last, there appeared to be too much focus on internal rather than external indicators.

As a result of these concerns, there have been multiple projects and articles. Ultimately Kaplan and Norton released their bestseller, *The Balanced Scorecard*.[2] A wide variety of Fortune 1000 firms and many other private sector firms around the world now use the Balanced Scorecard (BSC).

THE BALANCED SCORECARD FOR THE FEDERAL GOVERNMENT

This book is an attempt to improve the management of the federal government. It will show the relevance of the BSC to federal government organizations and how it can be effectively implemented to improve performance. The book will reflect "best practices" in BSC federal government implementation and present various federal organizations at different stages of implementation.

This book is about implementation. This book is about the requirements of the BSC and the benefits that can be obtained. It is about the differences and the similarities of implementing the BSC in the federal government and in the private sector.

However, the BSC is not a silver bullet. If the federal government's top management supports BSC implementation as they have supported initial GPRA efforts, progress will be slow in many federal organizations.

The BSC was developed with the private sector in mind, a place where the performance "bar" is somewhat higher and performance measurement more precise. Most federal government organizations do not have the luxury of daily, weekly, and monthly profit and loss (P&L) statements. Therefore, the crispness of the BSC gets a little "fuzzy" within the federal domain.

In the private sector BSC, vision and strategy drive operational action to satisfy four areas: (1) financial, (2) customer, (3) internal business process, and (4) learning and growth. Imme-

---

[2]Kaplan, Robert S., and David P. Norton, *The Balanced Scorecard*. Boston: Harvard Business School Press, 1996.

diately, issues of implementation and effectiveness emerge. In the private sector, if the firm is successful in the market, the customer is satisfied, and the financial returns are satisfactory, the firm will be successful and grow over time. In the federal arena, the amount of dollars authorized and appropriated each year has something to do with efficiency and effectiveness but also responds to the environment, politics, and other relevant issues.

It is clear that the BSC has the potential to make a contribution to federal government management. Federal government performance can be improved, but it will not be an easy task. Multiple GPRA implementation deficiencies need to be resolved. Top management must take the issues of mission, vision, and implementation as "their" responsibility and not delegate them down one or two levels. That also means that top management must be involved in routine reviews of progress against goals that show that the BSC is indeed a concept with "teeth, life, and support."

The next chapter of this book details how the BSC contributes to private sector management. The remainder of the book describes best practices in federal government departments and organizations.

WHY THIS TIME MAY BE DIFFERENT

It is possible that this time may indeed be different. The 7,000-member Senior Executive Service (SES) leads the 2-million member federal government workforce. The SES drives the federal government in its day-to-day operations and develops its long-range goals. Past SES performance has been measured in a variety of ways.

The June 21, 2000 *Federal Register* contained an item from the Office of Personnel Management.[3] Among other things, it proposes appraising senior executive performance using measures that balance organizational results with customer, employee, and other perspectives.

If these elite personnel are going to be graded annually on their performance on these Balanced Measures, this time they may pay more attention to the requirements of GPRA and the new process of strategic planning, performance planning, and performance reporting. Let us hope so.

---

[3]"Managing Senior Executive Performance." *Federal Register* 65, no. 120 (June 21, 2000): 38442.

CHAPTER 2

The Balanced Scorecard in the Private Sector: Measuring Business Strategy

Kaplan and Norton[1] deal with a number of important issues in their discussion of measuring business strategy. Their basic point is that to be successful in an increasingly competitive world, businesses must satisfy a variety of benchmarks, not just financial performance. They outline several perspectives that must be achieved, including a financial perspective, a customer perspective, an internal business perspective, and a learning and growth perspective.

FINANCIAL PERSPECTIVE

The financial perspective is key to the Balanced Scorecard (BSC) approach. In many ways, financial perspectives provide the focus for goals, objectives, and measures and indicators across the scorecard. For most commercial organizations, financial areas of decreasing cost, improving productivity, increasing revenue, enhancing effective asset utilization, and reducing risk provide the required linkage across all BSC perspectives.

Companies can choose from a variety of financial objectives, depending on the stage in their life cycle. Kaplan and Norton simplify the choices and identify three stages of the life cycle: (1) grow, (2) sustain, and (3) harvest. While these concepts are important in the private sector, they are less relevant in the public sector.

In the early stage of the private sector life cycle, commercial companies have products or services with large growth potential. To develop this potential, private sector organizations must invest in these products or services. Their objectives and measures will be tailored to such factors as growth rate percentages in revenue and sales growth rates in various targeted markets or customer groups.

Later in the private sector life cycle, business will be in the *sustain* stage. Most private sector companies are in this stage. Here the strategy of the company changes. In addition to concern about sales growth, firms need to be earning a good return on their invested capital.

Later in the private sector life cycle, firms will want to *harvest* investments made in the two earlier cycles. New investment will be curtailed except when necessary to maintain existing capabilities. Investment projects in this stage would require short-period paybacks and definite, less risky returns. Financial objectives would be operating cash flow (before depreciation) and working capital reductions.

Consequently, as the organization moves though the life cycle in the private sector, different financial performance is required. Financial measures change to align the interest of the shareholders and the investors with the reality of the marketplace to ensure that the firm provides the appropriate financial returns.

---

[1]Kaplan, Robert S., and David P. Norton. *The Balanced Scorecard*. Boston: Harvard Business School Press, 1996.

Kaplan and Norton show that three financial themes drive the strategies of grow, sustain, and harvest. The financial themes are (1) revenue growth and mix, (2) cost reduction/productivity improvement, and (3) asset utilization/investment strategy.

Revenue growth and mix refers to how the firm would expand the product and service offering to reach new customers and markets, and change the products and services toward higher value-added offerings. Measurement would include sales growth by business segment or percent revenue increase from new customers and new product or service offerings. In any theme or strategy, measurement should show what the firm is trying to achieve and then develop the most appropriate, most effective measures and indicators for that theme or strategy.

Cost reduction/productivity improvement refers to efforts to lower the direct costs of products or services and reduce indirect costs. One of the more manageable aspects of the private sector problem, as opposed to the federal government, is the ability to do, measure, and incentivize this behavior. Since the private sector is reporting and measuring these objectives on a daily, weekly, and monthly basis, progress may be much more achievable and measurable. The federal government not only lacks the system capability and the requirements to measure and report these indicators, but also may have political considerations relative to the issue that result in productivity improvement and cost reduction not being major program goals. The ability to apply some of the "best practices" from the private sector becomes more difficult in the federal arena.

The last theme—asset utilization/investment strategy—is also a more difficult one to implement in the federal government. In the private sector, firms strive to achieve higher utilization of their fixed asset base by using scarce resources more efficiently and getting rid of assets that provide inadequate returns. Through the ubiquitous financial controls and objectives, this is a normal way of doing business in the private sector. This approach is not so easily implemented in the federal government, where many disincentives may apply. As a recent example, Congress decided during the budget discussion for FY 2000 that 1 percent of the budget should be reduced to provide a method of reducing fraud, waste, and abuse in the execution of executive branch programs. How much of that 1 percent would have been covered if the various elected officials who have taken care of their constituents withdrew the obvious "pork" already in the budget?

Kaplan and Norton start with financial objectives, recognizing that the private sector firm must achieve above-average financial returns based on the capital invested or it will not exist in the long run. Interestingly, the private sector firm must effectively and efficiently use financial objectives and measures to drive its operations as the federal government has, in the past, been required to spend the budget dollars appropriated and authorized. This federal government requirement has resulted in less than effective and efficient utilization of those dollars. The GPRA requirement mandates that those financial assets be turned into appropriate results across the country.

Financial objectives and measures will continue to increase in importance in the federal government as positive steps are taken to make the federal government more businesslike. However, it will be a difficult task to move government to results-oriented activity rather than a "budget driven/spend your funds to get more" approach.

CUSTOMER PERSPECTIVE

In the customer perspective, the private sector company must identify the customer and in what segment it will compete. These customers and these segments must then deliver the financial results necessary to sustain the business. The customer perspective allows the private sector company to align core customer outcomes such as satisfaction, loyalty, acquisition, retention, and profitability. It also allows the company to measure explicitly the value proposition that the company offers the customer and the segments that it has targeted. Value propositions are the drivers of the core customer outcomes.

Core measurement outcomes are generic across all kinds of organizations. They include measures of (1) market share, (2) customer retention, (3) customer acquisition, (4) customer satisfaction, and (5) customer profitability.

The customer value proposition represents the attributes that private sector companies provide through their products and services. These value propositions create loyalty and satisfaction in the targeted customer segments of the market. Value propositions will vary across different industries and across different segments of various industries. However, Kaplan and Norton noticed a common set of attributes across the industries within which they have worked on the Balanced Scorecard. These three categories of attributes are (1) product /service attributes, (2) customer relationship, and (3) image and reputation.

Product/service attributes relate to the functionality of the product or service and its price and quality. Some customers want consistently low-cost products while other customers are willing to pay for unique products, services, and quality. The customer approach chosen must be able to provide the financial returns necessary to build and sustain the business over time by yielding a sufficient return on investment assets utilized.

Customer relationship concerns elements such as delivering the product or service to the customer and measuring such things as how responsive the company is and what the time of that response is. It also includes how the customer feels about dealing with the firm. What kind of employees do you want dealing with the customer? How knowledgeable are they? How does the customer feel about the level of service provided by the company? How responsive is the company initially in regular times, and how does it respond when there is a problem? Is there convenient access to the product and service provided by the company? More and more companies today are providing 7×24 service in a variety of industries.

Image and reputation deal with those intangible factors that attract customers to various firms in the private sector. Firms are able to generate customer loyalty beyond the tangible aspects of the products and services provided to the customer. A good example of this concept is the high level of product and service accompanied by a variety of aligned policies that state that the customer is always right. Nordstrom customer service is legendary, and the loyalty of its customers is a vital part of its corporate strategy.

A set of core outcome measures should be developed that target the customer and his or her relationship to the private sector company directly. The product and service delivery should be measured on functionality, quality, and price. The relationship with the customer should be measured on the quality of the purchasing experience and the personal relationship of that experience. Last, the image and reputation of the firm should be developed to strengthen the execution of the strategy in the market and the market segment that has been targeted.

INTERNAL BUSINESS PERSPECTIVE

Internal business perspective means that the firm must identify those processes that are most critical to achieving success. Thus, this analysis must target those processes that are most critical to achieving shareholder and customer objectives. Kaplan and Norton state that this analysis should be conducted as an internal value chain analysis. They start with the front end—the innovation process. Firms start with customers' needs and then develop new products and solutions that will be offered to customers to satisfy those needs. Next they look at the operating process whereby the firm delivers products and services to the customers of the firm. They finish with the post-sale service offering that adds value to the products and services sold to customers to satisfy their needs.

This focus on the internal business process and the derivation of objectives and measures is one of the most distinctive differences between the Balanced Scorecard and more traditional performance measurement systems. Traditional systems rely more on financial measures and on controlling and improving existing departments and divisions. The BSC puts more emphasis on improvement of the operation as a whole and the integration of results that will achieve both stockholder and customer objectives. This integration direction will be extremely helpful in the federal government where some of the most "ineffective, moat-like silos" exist. There are few incentives in many government operations to drive integration of action for results that will support the customer and the taxpayer rather than support the entrenched incumbents in government operations.

Kaplan and Norton note that all companies are attempting to reduce cycle times, improve quality, maximize throughput, increase yields, and lower costs for their business processes. Therefore, in the private sector this push for improved performance will not necessarily lead to a unique strategy. However, in the federal government this push for performance is not as widespread. Various federal agencies could provide unique contributions to their customers and to the taxpayers by setting objectives and measures in the five areas mentioned above. In fact, there are few federal agencies or departments that should not be doing so.

LEARNING AND GROWTH PERSPECTIVE

The final perspective develops objectives, measures, and indicators to drive organizational learning and growth. Objectives in this perspective provide the foundation to enable objectives in the other three perspectives to be achieved. It is not unusual to find many private sector organizations where it is difficult to invest in the enhancement of employees, processes, and systems. This is particularly true when too much emphasis is placed on short-term financial performance. These investments are usually expensed; therefore, cutbacks in these expenses are a quick way to get a short-term "pop" in earnings. Managers with a short-term outlook hope that this misallocation of short-term investments that flow to the bottom line do not catch up with them before they leave. If the right level of emphasis on investments and attention is not provided to your people, processes, and systems, the downside impact will be felt. This is particularly true in the public sector where insufficient funds are frequently allocated for personal and professional development of the workforce and the negative consequences are seen routinely across the federal government.

Kaplan and Norton identify three principal categories for the learning and growth perspective across a wide variety of private sector firms: (1) employee capabilities; (2) information system capabilities; and (3) motivation, empowerment, and alignment.

Employee Capabilities

One of the biggest changes in the past 10 to 20 years involves employee contributions to organizations. Successful organizations require continual improvement over time. Many tasks that were previously assigned to employees have been automated. Jobs that previously were narrow and uncomplicated have given way to automated ways to accomplish that work. Today's employees are consistently asked to do more and think about how they can continually improve their performance and the performance of their work group. This change places more responsibility on the individual employee and his or her capacity to think and respond to a variety of job requirements.

This shift in job requirements demands a change in employees to ensure that their minds and creative abilities are directed and aligned with the objectives of the organization. This will be a particularly important factor in implementing the BSC in the public sector since this transition of employee responsibilities and tasks has occurred but the requisite actions and investments by the public sector organizations have not always accompanied this transition.

Three core employee measurements include (1) employee satisfaction, (2) employee retention, and (3) employee productivity. These measures loomed even more important as the 20th century wound down with some of the lowest unemployment rates in the United States in the past several decades. Private sector employees in many fields and in many geographic areas had wide choices and opportunities for employment. Therefore, these three employee measures became even more critical in many industries.

Employee satisfaction can be measured in surveys conducted annually or on some other schedule. These surveys might address factors such as: (1) job recognition, (2) sufficient access to information, (3) appropriate involvement in decisions, (4) encouragement to be creative and innovative, (5) sufficient staff support, and (6) overall satisfaction with the company.

Employee retention is an increasingly important issue as firms move away from manufacturing to service industries. As the individual is asked to be more creative and deal with more thoughtful, innovative situations, the value of the long-term investment in the employee becomes clear. As the business world develops the concept of knowledge management, much of that asset is what the human component of the organization has learned and passed on for the organization to improve its performance and increase its shareholder value in the future. If organizations do not retain the employees they need to be successful, future success will be more difficult. Moreover, adequate financial returns to the shareholder, and product and service returns to the customer, will be more difficult to achieve.

Employee productivity can be measured in a variety of ways. One of the simplest measures is revenue per employee. However, revenue can increase while the return to invested assets goes down. Therefore, one might measure profit or earnings before interest and taxes (EBIT) per employee as a more appropriate indicator. Employee productivity needs to be measured in ways that are integrated with the key factors of success across the organization even as the organizational environment changes the challenges to the organization.

If the employees of an organization need to be re-skilled, then specific drivers of learning and growth involve staff competencies, the technology infrastructure, and the climate for action in the organization.

Information System Capabilities

Information system capabilities may be one of the most important factors in this system of objectives and measures. Employee motivation and skills are important for high-performance organizations providing substantial returns to shareholders and customers, but they are probably not sufficient in this day and age. Effective employees in this increasingly competitive environment must have fast, accurate information on products and services, on internal business processes, and on the financial consequences of their individual decisions. With the increasing competitiveness of the environment and the growing demands of customers to reduce cost, increase quality, minimize cycle time, and enhance customer satisfaction, many firms will fail or achieve minimal success due to the problems in information systems. Some private sector companies have developed objectives and measures focused on a strategic information coverage ratio. These measures of strategic information availability look at the percentage of processes with real-time quality, cycle time, and cost feedback available, and the percentage of customer-facing employees with on-line customer information.

Motivation, Empowerment, and Alignment

Kaplan and Norton suggest a number of measures that can be used in the area of motivation, empowerment, and alignment. They can vary from a simple measure (e.g., the number of suggestions per employee) to a more complex measure (e.g., the number of suggestions implemented) to an even more complex measure that quantifies process improvements (e.g., quality, time, and performance).

Performance drivers for individual and organizational alignment focus on the alignment between company and individuals/departments. This alignment is critical throughout the organization to ensure that the right objectives are achieved. When this alignment is checked throughout the organization, the element of team performance must be effectively addressed. Kaplan and Norton reference a variety of measures for team building and team performance in addition to measures for individual performance.

Kaplan and Norton note that there are fewer examples of measures in the learning and growth perspective because many companies have not yet started to develop them. Companies do not appear to be linking the learning and growth area to their strategy and long-term objectives, and instead assume that the outcomes of these efforts are correct and ends in themselves. This is a good area for federal government analysis and experimentation since the long-term efficacy of the federal workforce and its information technology systems are key to effective government now and in the future.

CONCLUSION

Kaplan and Norton make several key points in their wrap-up on measuring business strategy. First, they note that their comments relate to an organizational unit in the private sector called a strategic business unit. These units are generally much smaller and less complex than the agencies and departments of the federal government. Therefore, their BSC comments have to be carefully considered and not applied arbitrarily.

Second, a successful BSC is one that communicates a strategy through an integrated set of measurements that includes both financial and non-financial items. The federal government can use this effectively, but the concept of strategy is not one that is used or understood throughout the federal government. A large, long-term training effort will be required to derive the benefits of the BSC.

Third, the BSC needs to be linked to the organizational strategy by three principles: (1) cause-and-effect relationship, (2) performance driver, and (3) financials. Moreover, the outcome and performance driver measures on the balanced scorecard must result from intensive and broad-based discussions between senior- and mid-level management.

Fourth, the best BSCs are those that allow development of the underlying strategy of the business unit from the listing of objectives and measures and the associated linkages among them. Last, the use of the BSC to develop corporate strategy as distinguished from strategic business unit strategy is in the early development stage. Over time, more research information will be available in this complex area.

The Kaplan and Norton text contains many detailed examples explaining how various private sector companies have employed the BSC concept. The book does not delve deeply into particulars but provides the reader with sufficient detail to explore the BSC in more depth.

CHAPTER 3

The Balanced Scorecard at the Federal Aviation Administration Logistics Center

The Federal Aviation Administration Logistics Center (FAALC) in Oklahoma City provides one of the best organizational examples of the effective use of the BSC over a period of years. This chapter first details how the organization dealt with strategy in the 1993 to 1994 period. It then recounts how the BSC was discovered and used in the strategic plan published in 1997. Last, it demonstrates how the strategic plan for 1999 through 2002 reflects even more maturity in the use of the BSC.

Some of this material can viewed on the FAALC Web site (www.bts.gov/ntl/data/ strateg.pdf). For those with more detailed questions, Sheree VanNoy, the FAALC strategic planning coordinator since 1993, has generously offered to answer questions by telephone (405-954-0421).

FAALC STRATEGIC PLAN FOR 1994

The material that follows is adapted from the Federal Aviation Administration Logistics Center, *Strategic Planning, Vision of the Future,* August 1992. It reflects how FAALC's 1994 plan dealt with strategy at much too high a level to drive day-to-day performance. One section of the 1994 plan follows; another portion is presented in Appendix A.

INTRODUCTION

"Nine tenths of wisdom consists of being wise in time."
"Keep your eyes on the stars; keep your feet on the ground."
—Theodore Roosevelt

Theodore Roosevelt spoke the words above around the beginning of the twentieth century at a time when this country was experiencing enormous changes associated with the industrial revolution. Mr. Roosevelt himself is credited with one of the most remarkable and foresighted accomplishments in the history of America, building the Panama Canal. Undoubtedly, his successes during those times of rapid change can be attributed to the philosophy embodied in these statements.

Just as during Teddy Roosevelt's lifetime, we are witnessing rapid social, economic, political, and technological changes. New and improved technology, the availability of information, and a new global economy are a few of the factors driving changes in the aviation system. Changes in management philosophy, increased public interest in how tax dollars are being used, and cultural diversity are factors driving the "reinvention" of government. All of these changes and other factors will influence the future of the FAA and the FAA Logistics Center.

Our guiding vision is to be the preferred choice throughout the FAA and non-FAA organizations for logistics support of the National Airspace System. The changes we face may present either an opportunity or a threat to making that vision a reality. The more eminent the change the greater likelihood the change will be a threat. On the other hand, given time to prepare and plan for a change we can often create an opportunity for growth or improvement. Through the strategic planning process we can stay in touch with those changes which will influence our future, anticipate the impact of those changes, and build a set of strategies to ensure the changes we face present opportunities which support our vision.

This publication summarizes the results of the FAALC strategic planning efforts to date. This version is provided for internal use by the FAALC employees in order to document the strategic planning process and publicize the FAALC management team's view of the future and strategies for meeting the challenges of the future. As we continue in the implementation of this plan we will learn more and develop a clearer picture of the future. Our strategic plan will be adjusted accordingly. This plan should, therefore, be viewed as a living document, growing, evolving, and changing, as we continue to gather information.

PART I

Strategic Plan Summary

I. Purpose: The FAALC strategic plan provides a direction for the future based on analysis of factors that will affect current FAALC business operations.

II. Process: FAALC management team analyzed current environment, external factors that could change the environment, projected how the FAALC will look in the future, and identified strategies to meet challenges of the future. Employees will take a more active role in development of action plans and implementation.

III. Key Elements of the Plan:
A. Major Factors Affecting the Future
   1. Replacement of traditional ground based systems by Global Positioning Satellite (GPS). GPS will mean less hardware in the field = reduction in required depot level support.
   2. Increased use of Non-developmental Items (NDI) and Commercial Off-the-Shelf (COTS) equipment and systems. NDI/COTS means more contractor support for field maintenance.
C. FAALC Vision: The FAALC is the preferred choice for logistics support to the NAS. Our strategy is to remain a viable, cost effective part of the FAA.
D. Key Issue Areas Addressed in Future Business Model
   1. NAS Logistics Support in FAA
      a. Current: Decentralized functions. Numerous FAA activities have some responsibility.
      b. Future: Integrated—Life Cycle Management common goal/mission of various players.
   2. FAALC Mission
      a. Current: Depot Level Supply Support—Equipment focus.
      b. Future: Life Cycle Management Support—System focus.
   3. FAALC Customers
      a. Current: AAF, AVN, MMAC, AXA, other government agencies, international.
      b. Future: Same basic customers, expanded partnerships.
   4. Lines of Business—In the future we will assume new lines of business. We will continue to perform current lines of business but there will be changes.

    5. Resources (Financial)
       a. Current: Fragmented budget process.
       b. Future: Life Cycle Management budget process. Our funds based on ability to "sell" our products and services.
    6. People
       a. Current: Specialized skills, functional focus.
       b. Future: Multi-skilled, product team focus.
    7. Organization
       a. Current: Functional alignment "stovepipe."
       b. Future: Product/service alignment, fewer layers, team concept.
  E. Primary Strategies—"The Foundation of the Strategic Plan"
    1. Streamline Current Operations—Improve processes, customer service.
    2. Increase Competitiveness—Become cost conscious, improve productivity, prepare to compete with contractors for maintenance on systems.
    3. Enter New Lines of Business—Management of AF Field level contracts, Centralized Field level maintenance, Configuration Management, National Logistics Information Service.
    4. Utilize New Business Method—Life Cycle Management
  F. Summary: We can meet challenges of the future through teamwork and maximum utilization of our knowledge, skills, abilities, and experience.

PART 2

Designing Our Future—"The Process"

The FAALC Management Team began the strategic planning process in November 1992 by planning to plan and outlining a strategic planning process. Since that time the process has evolved as the team and its understanding of the potential changes in the FAA has matured. In simple terms the process utilized consists of six major steps:

1. Describing our current situation—Where we are today?
2. Painting a picture of where we want to be in the future
3. Identifying the "gaps" between "today" and "tomorrow"—What is different between our picture of today and tomorrow?
4. Mapping out broad strategies to bridge the gaps—How (in very broad terms) can the FAALC get to tomorrow?
5. Developing action plans to accomplish strategies—Specifically what steps should we take, who will lead the effort, when will it be accomplished?
6. Implement the action plans, track progress, measure results, and adjust gaps as necessary.

There are numerous steps that must be taken within each phase of the strategic planning process we have described, as well as a great deal of information to be considered. Figure 3–1 provides a diagram of the strategic planning process utilized by the FAALC management team. A more detailed discussion of each step follows Figure 3–1.

The FAALC management team has completed the first four steps in the process. The result of this first strategic planning cycle is summarized in this document.

A number of employees have already been involved in initiatives which grew out of the strategic planning process. However, we are now ready to enter the Action Plan and Implementation phases of the process on a broader, more structured basis.

Process Discussion

1. **Environmental Assessment**—The process of describing our current situation and identifying possible factors that may influence our future. Identification of mandates, defining our mission and organizational values, conducting an external and internal scan are part of the environmental assessment.

   a. Mandates—Laws, orders, policies, agreements, or commitments that set a boundary on what you can do now and in the future.

   b. Mission/Value—Purpose of the organization and the operating values that the organization will use.

   c. Internal Scan—The process of identifying what resources we have available to shape our future.

   d. External Scan—The process of identifying those forces acting on the FAALC from the outside. Primary focus is on identifying any opportunities that will exist and any threats to the FAALC current operations. Information is gathered from customers, suppliers, and other stakeholders regarding their expectations. The FAA Strategic Plan, our key stakeholders' strategic plans, and political, economic, social and technological trends also provide critical information.

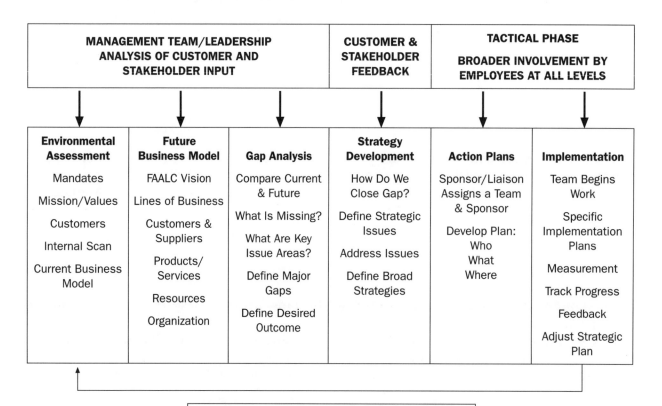

Figure 3–1. Strategic Planning Process. *Source:* Adapted from Federal Aviation Administration Logistics Center, *Strategic Planning, Vision of the Future,* August 1992.

e. Current Business Model—A description of the key elements of our current business model, i.e., how we do business today. The key elements were identified as NAS Logistics Support in the FAA, the FAALC mission, Customers, Lines of Business, Resources, People and Organization. This is based on information gathered in the Environmental Assessment, and analysis of that information.

2. **Future Business Model**—Describes the FAALC Vision of the Future. Includes a statement, which describes the direction of the FAALC that indicates success in accomplishing our mission in the future. We also describe our future lines of business, the customer base served by that line of business, and the products and/or services provided to that customer. For comparison purposes the key elements defined in the Future Business Model were the same as those defined in the Current Business Model. This is based on analysis of information gathered in the environmental assessment.

3. **Gap Analysis**—During this step in the process we compare our current situation to our overall vision for the FAALC. The framework for accomplishing this is comparison of the current business model to the future business model. By systematically comparing each key element of the current and future business models we discuss the differences, identify potential issues or problems, and finally identify the major gap areas which must be closed to get to our future business model. In our analysis there was a major gap in each of the seven key elements of the model, these then became the key issue areas used to focus our strategy development.

4. **Strategy Development**—At this step we define in very broad terms how the FAALC can achieve the model of the future. First we write a vision for each of the major gaps, i.e., what the FAALC will do, how it will operate, or what characteristic will change if the gap is closed. We also define key strategic issues that must be addressed or considered in the action plans. This will serve as the ultimate goal for the team, or teams, assigned to work this gap.

5. **Action Plan (or Strategy Prospectus) Development**—The development of action plans marks the initial transition of the strategic plan to tactical or operational planning and implementation. This step requires broader employee and management participation. Sponsorship for each major gap is assigned to a member of the management team. In some cases sponsorship may be shared between two members. The sponsor is responsible to establish a team of FAALC employees to begin studying the major gap and develop an action plan. The information generated by the management team through the first four steps will be provided to each team, along with any additional guidance the sponsor deems appropriate. This information is provided in what is referred to as a "Strategy Prospectus." Teams will typically be comprised of employees from various functional areas, i.e., different AML Divisions, and may require membership from outside the FAALC depending on the nature of the assignment. Action plans will outline primary goals and objectives that must be accomplished to realize the vision of the closed gap, and a timetable for accomplishing these goals. Additional "sub-teams" may be required to work specific goals and objectives.

6. **Implementation**—At this step the management team begins to track and monitor the implementation of the Action Plans. Additional or new information may be gained during this phase which will necessitate adjustment to the future business model, may change the nature of focus of a gap, point to a new gap, or require new priorities be placed on action plans.

FAALC STRATEGIC PLAN FOR 1997

Much positive change is evident In the FAALC 1997 strategic plan. The BSC is implemented through four different areas: (1) the customer perspective, (2) the financial stakeholder perspective, (3) the internal business perspective, and (4) the learning and innovation perspective. These areas are laid out as several strategic goals in each perspective into several measures in each perspective and finally into multiple targets in each perspective. This allows the plan to be driven throughout the organization in order to implement the organization strategy effectively.

The following material is adapted from the Federal Aviation Administration Logistics Center, *Strategic Plan: Our Guide to the Future,* 1997.

Introduction

Purpose

The FAA Logistics Center's strategic plan provides a direction for the future based on analysis of factors affecting current Logistics Center business operations.

Process

A group comprised of Logistics Center managers, labor representatives, and employees projected how the Logistics Center will look in the future. The FAA Logistics Center management team analyzed the current environment, external factors that could change that environment, and identified strategies to meet future challenges.

In March 1997, the strategic planning group revised the strategic goals and applied the "Balanced Scorecard Approach" to develop measures and targets for each strategic goal.

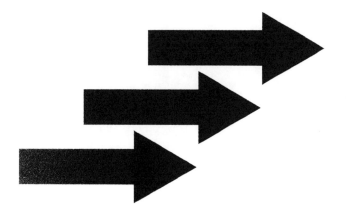

1

Environmental Assessment

"The National Performance Review is about change -- historic change -- in the way government works." This is the first line of "From Red Tape to Results, Creating a Government that Works Better and Costs Less, Report of the National Performance Review," published in September 1993. The FAA Logistics Center's strategic planning group not only sees change in our future, but wants to lead the way in making historic changes in the way we work.

The following factors are some of the most significant changes affecting our future:

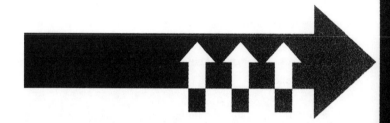

Major Factors Affecting the Future

- Replacement of traditional ground-based systems by Global Positioning System (GPS).

- Increased use of non-developmental items and commercial off-the-shelf (COTS) equipment and systems.

- The National Performance Review — a challenge to create a government that works better and costs less.

- New flexibility in the areas of human resource management and acquisition.

- Increased competition for shrinking budget allocations.

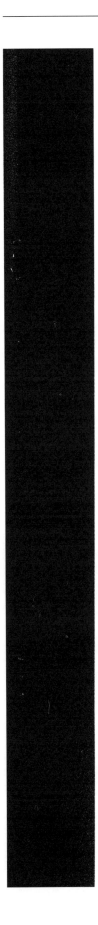

Vision

The FAA Logistics Center is a world-class, customer-driven logistics organization whose quality services are in demand throughout the FAA and worldwide.

Mission

The FAA Logistics Center provides comprehensive logistics support and high quality products, assuring safety of the flying public, and satisfies the needs of the National Airspace System (NAS) and other valued customers.

Key Business Processes

Key business processes are those processes cutting across FAA Logistics Center divisional or functional lines. All Logistics Center employees play a role in delivering products or services produced by one or more of these processes.

- Contractor Maintenance Logistics Support (CMLS)
- Contractor Depot Logistics Support (CDLS)
- Organic logistics support
- Site depot services
- Acquisition planning
- Refurbishment

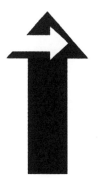

3

Organizational Values

We Believe In and Are Committed To...

- Customer and Employee Satisfaction

- Quality and Teamwork

- Leadership and Communications

- Loyalty, Commitment, and Trust

- Diversity and Corporate Citizenship

- Innovation and Risk-Taking

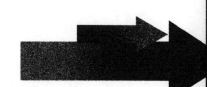

Organizational Values Will Be Achieved Because Our Culture Says...

- Everyone understands the vision and priorities of the organization.

- People enjoy coming to work and take pride in their job.

- Everyone is treated with respect.

- Leaders model the value of employee involvement and customer satisfaction.

- People are committed and loyal to this organization.

- Everyone knows their customers and their needs.

- People have the opportunity to influence how the work is done.

- We know and measure how well we're doing in satisfying customers.

- Ideas are exchanged openly.

- We systematically analyze and improve how the work is done.

- Decisions are usually made by consensus.

4

Strategies

The FAA Logistics Center will employ two broad strategies to achieve our vision:

- Focus on the customer to become a customer-driven organization.

- Increase and/or sustain business for the FAA Logistics Center.

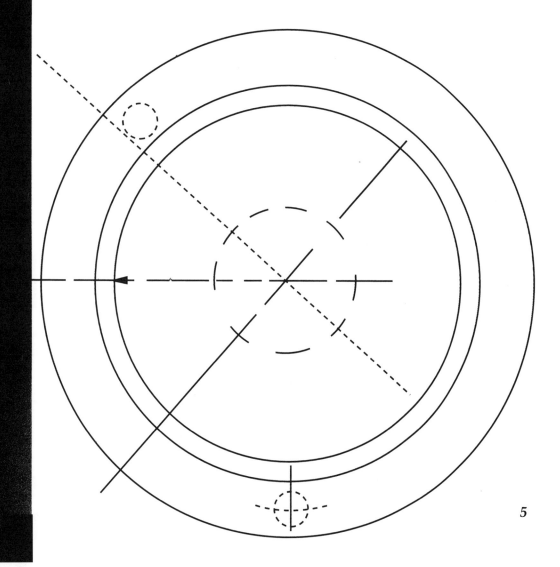

5

Strategic Goals, Measures, & Targets

The FAA Logistics Center's strategic goals, measures and targets were developed using the "Balanced Scorecard Approach." The Balanced Scorecard Approach says the success of an organization is dependent upon balancing various aspects of the organization to achieve overall success. Managers must look at the organization from four basic perspectives:

- **The Customer Perspective** - What must we do to satisfy, retain, and attract new customers?

- **The Financial Stakeholder Perspective -** What must we do to increase business and ensure financial success?

- **The Internal Business Perspective -** What internal processes must we excel at to satisfy our customers and assure financial success?

- **The Learning and Innovation Perspective -** What must we do to develop employee skills and technology to continue adding value to our customers and improve our capabilities?

The FAA Logistics Center's **Balanced Scorecard** consists of the following:

- **Strategic goals** translate our broad strategies into actionable goals to achieve our vision of the future.

- **Measures** describe what we will measure to determine whether or not we have met our goals.

- **Targets** for the measures are set 3 to 5 years out and are designed to s-t-r-e-t-c-h our performance. If we achieve these targets, we will transform the FAA Logistics Center and achieve our vision.

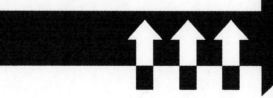

The FAA Logistics Center's Strategy

To achieve the **FAA Logistics Center's** vision, we have two broad strategies. These are to be "customer driven" and to "increase or sustain business for the Logistics Center." These two strategies must be balanced. Our financial stakeholders influence our ability to increase our business. We must balance their requirements with our customers' needs and expectations. The following diagram shows the **FAA Logistics Center's** strategic goals established to provide this balance.

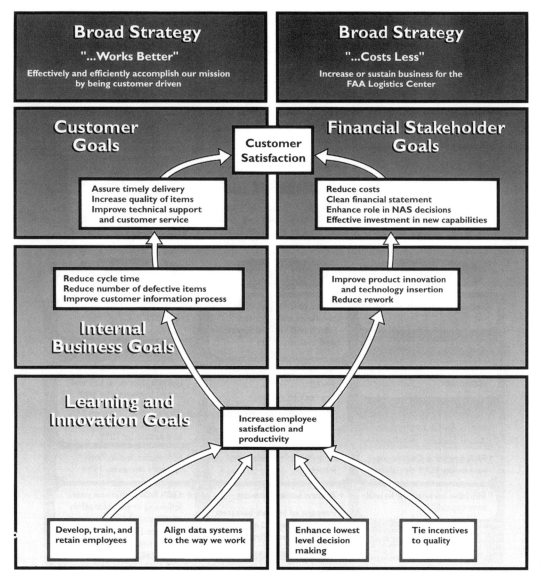

Broad Strategy

"...Works Better"

Effectively and efficiently accomplish our mission by being customer driven

Broad Strategy

"...Costs Less"

Increase or sustain business for the FAA Logistics Center

Customer Goals

Customer Satisfaction

Assure timely delivery
Increase quality of items
Improve technical support and customer service

Financial Stakeholder Goals

Reduce costs
Clean financial statement
Enhance role in NAS decisions
Effective investment in new capabilities

Reduce cycle time
Reduce number of defective items
Improve customer information process

Improve product innovation and technology insertion
Reduce rework

Internal Business Goals

Learning and Innovation Goals

Increase employee satisfaction and productivity

Develop, train, and retain employees

Align data systems to the way we work

Enhance lowest level decision making

Tie incentives to quality

7

THE CUSTOMER PERSPECTIVE

STRATEGIC GOAL	MEASURE	TARGET
• Increase customer satisfaction	• Customer satisfaction rating	• Improve overall rating to max rating in 90% of categories by end of 1999
• Assure timely delivery	• Percent of on-time deliveries as defined by customer	• 100% on-time by end of 1999
• Increase quality of items delivered	• Percent of defective shipments (product defective) • Percent of defective shipments (quantity, pkg, marking, or wrong item basis for defective shipment)	• Zero defective shipments by end of 1999
• Increase quality of technical support and customer service	• # of customer queries satisfied the first time • # of customer complaints regarding technical support and customer service	• Increase from current to 100% by end of 1999 • Zero by end of 1999

THE FINANCIAL STAKEHOLDER PERSPECTIVE

STRATEGIC GOAL	MEASURE	TARGET
• Reduce cost	• Average unit cost of products and services which will include direct and indirect costs	• 30% Reduction in unit cost by 2001
• Produce clean financial statement	• Clean assessment by 3rd party • Percent of variance between DAFIS, LIS, and actual inventory value	• Less than 5% variance in quantity between LIS and actual inventory by 9/97 • 0% variance between LIS, agency accounting system, and actual by 1999
• FAA Logistics Center plays role in key NAS decisions	• Number of non-support issues	• 50% reduction in non-support issues by 1999
• Effective investment to add new capabilities	• Return on investment • Percent of budget invested in human capital and capital improvements	• 150% ROI within one year following implementation of new capability • Allocate 15% of budget to capital improvement by 2001

THE INTERNAL BUSINESS PERSPECTIVE

STRATEGIC GOAL	MEASURE	TARGET
• Reduce cycle time	• Cycle time	• 50% reduction in cycle time by 1999
• Improve product delivery time	• Delivery time (incrementally)	• Delivery in 6 hours by 1999
• Reduce rework	• Percent of items reworked	• .00001% of items reworked by 1999
• Reduce number of defective items received	• Number of discrepant items received	• One complaint per 10,000 received by 1999
• Improve product innovation and technology insertion	• Number of NSN's that are support condition red	• 75% reduction by 1999
• Improve process for customer information	• Customer satisfaction survey	• Overall customer rating in this category of 4 or higher (scale of 1-5) by 1999

THE LEARNING AND INNOVATION PERSPECTIVE

STRATEGIC GOAL	MEASURE	TARGET
• Develop, train, retain current workers. Attract, develop, and retain knowledge workers	• Employee skills assessment	• Complimentary mix with broad-based knowledge and technical skills
• Align data systems to the way we work to meet employee and customer needs	• User satisfaction survey • System access availability time	• Survey indicates average rating of 4 or higher (scale of 1-5) in this category by 1999 • 75% improvement in system availability time by 1999
• Tie incentives to quality	• Percent of employee awards related to quality • Number of quality award nominations	• 50% increase in number of awards related to quality by 1999 • Achieve DOT Quality Award by 1999, 3rd place for Baldrige by 2000
• Enhance lowest level decision-making	• Employee satisfaction/ organization climate survey • Leadership skills assessment	• Survey and assessment indicates 100% of assessed leaders' performance above satisfactory in this category by 1999

FAALC STRATEGIC PLAN FOR 1999–2002

The 1999–2002 strategic plan is yet another refinement on the application of the BSC. This plan lays out multiple strategic objectives for each Balanced Scorecard perspective followed by multiple measures and targets for each perspective.

The following material is adapted from the Federal Aviation Administration Logistics Center, *Strategic Plan: Our Guide to the Future: 1999–2002,* Oklahoma City, Oklahoma, FAA Information Media Division.

Introduction

Purpose

The Federal Aviation Administration Logistics Center (FAALC) strategic plan describes the strategic direction and business focus for the next 2 to 3 years. The Logistics Center is organizationally aligned under the Mike Monroney Aeronautical Center and the Assistant Administrator for Region and Center Operations within the FAA. As is the case with many organizations that are part of a larger government Agency, strategic priorities may change with little notice due to factors beyond our control or influence. Envisioning the future is never easy, however, under these circumstances it is particularly challenging. Our planning horizon was by necessity shorter than most strategic plans, and the plan is subject to change or modification in the near term.

Process

Consistent with our commitment to continuous improvement in all areas of the FAA Logistics Center, the strategic planning process was modified with the objective of enhancing the usefulness of this plan. The primary planning team, comprised of the senior managers, mid-level supervisors, and non-supervisory employees, commissioned a planning support team to conduct pre-planning research and analysis and revise the planning process. The planning support team membership included managers and staff support personnel. The support team reviewed the FAA Strategic Plan, primary customers' strategic plans, and even some potential competitors' strategic plans to assess external factors and ensure consistency with the Agency's strategic direction. A comprehensive analysis of future workload demand, completed by the FAALC Business Systems Group, was used extensively by the support group to predict future markets for Logistics Center services.

The support group also gathered feedback from internal users of the strategic plan. The feedback identified gaps in the previous plan that, if filled, would improve the plan's value as a framework for supplemental business plans developed by the FAALC divisions, groups, and teams. As a result new concepts, such as the "Strategy Statement," are included in this version. A "Supplemental Strategic Guide" is being published. The supplement is intended primarily for internal use and contains background information, definitions, explanations, and other information useful to the FAALC employees as they develop business plans in support of this plan.

Vision

The FAA Logistic Center is a world-class customer-driven organization whose quality services are in demand throughout the FAA and worldwide.

Mission

The FAALC ensures the safety of the flying public by providing material support, high quality electronic equipment repair, engineering services, inventory management, and other related services for the National Airspace System (NAS) and other valued customers.

How We Accomplish Our Mission

The FAALC is organizationally aligned by product lines and major support services. Each division is essentially a distinct business unit, capable of providing end-to-end services to a specific customer or segment of customers. The internal support functions are called systems groups. All divisions and groups report directly to the Logistics Center Program Director.

Business Units

Product Divisions

- Radar Products Division

- Communications Products Division

- Automation Products Division

- Navigation Landing and Weather Products Division

- Aircraft Products Division

Service Divisions

- Distribution Services Division

- Product Services Division

Support Groups

The primary mission of the support groups is to provide business services and related support to the business units, however, they may have some functions that are self-sustaining business operations.

· Business Systems Group

· Information Systems Group

· Quality Systems Group

Key Business Processes

Each business unit performs one or more of the key processes itemized below. These processes singularly, or in combination with others, are the key processes required to deliver products or services to our customers.

· Repair, fabrication, and overhaul of NAS equipment and systems which includes both centralized repair and site overhaul, as the customer requests

· Storage, distribution, and transportation of NAS parts and supplies

· Consulting services

  · Technical consulting services related to sustainment of NAS systems and equipment

  · Life cycle planning consulting services related to acquisition, supply support, maintenance, and decommissioning

· Inventory management

Organizational Values

We Believe In and Are Committed To...

- Customer and Employee Satisfaction

- Quality and Teamwork

- Leadership and Communications

- Loyalty, Commitment, and Trust

- Diversity and Corporate Citizenship

- Innovation and Risk-Taking

- Best Value Support for our Customers

Organizational Values Will Be Achieved Because Our Culture Says...

- Everyone understands the vision and priorities of the organization.

- People enjoy coming to work and take pride in the job they do.

- Everyone is treated with respect.

- Leaders model the value of employee involvement and customer satisfaction.

- People are committed and loyal to this organization.

- Everyone knows who their customers are and their needs.

- Everyone has the opportunity to influence how the work is done and what it costs.

- We know and measure how well we are doing in satisfying customers.

- Ideas are exchanged openly.

- We systematically analyze and improve how the work is done.

- Decisions are usually made by consensus.

Assumptions

This strategic plan is predicated on the following assumptions:

- The FAA Logistics Center will receive authorization to operate under a franchise fund during FY-2001.

- The FAA, and specifically Airway Facilities, will continue to be our primary customer.

- The FAA modernization program will retain some ground based navigation systems.

Environmental Assessment

Major Factors Affecting the Future

- FAA modernization including a phased replacement of many traditional ground based navigation systems by Global Positioning Satellite (GPS)

- The need for FAA to operate as a business and our responsibility to give the American public the best value for their dollar

- Customer behavior changes in a fee-for-service or similar environment

Strategies

The FAALC will employ three key strategies to achieve our vision, and position the Logistics Center for future success:

- Position the FAALC to rapidly respond to new customer demands by improving the flexibility and versatility of the organization.

- Work with agency product teams and the private sector to lower the cost of system ownership for our customers.

- Establish the FAALC as the fastest delivery source of quality products in the government sector.

Strategy Statement

Background

The FAALC Strategy Statement is a new feature of our strategic plan. It is included in response to feedback from our workforce. The strategic plan is intended as a tool to guide managers, supervisors, and employees throughout the organization in making business and operational decisions. Feedback regarding the previous plan indicated the plan would be a more useful tool if the Vision and Mission Statements were supplemented by clarifying the Logistics Center's strategic focus, or more clearly describing our direction. The Vision Statement clearly defines our key characteristics and how we want to be viewed by our customers and external stakeholders. The Mission statement describes in broad terms our primary function and ultimate responsibility. Both are necessary segments of our plan and serve to frame the picture of our future. However, a clear picture of what the FAALC will be is necessary for the plan to provide maximum value as a guide to our workforce. The strategy statement is intended to fill this gap.

Our objective is for the workforce to be able to know our strategy and use it as they would any other tool at their disposal.

FAALC Strategy Statement

The FAALC will continue to provide logistics support to our customers, and our primary thrust will continue to be the repair and distribution of NAS equipment and systems.

Our business focus for the near future will be on positioning the FAALC for rapid response to new customer demands, working to reduce the cost of system ownership for the FAA and other customers, and taking action to provide faster delivery service.

Each focus area has common strategic themes, specifically, growth and expansion of the Logistics Center's capabilities and business activities, achievement of operational excellence, and providing value to the customer.

We will constantly seek to improve the quality of our products and services, and be alert to new business opportunities that will add value to the service we provide to our primary customer, the FAA, and ultimately the flying public. We will demonstrate our pride and commitment as public servants dedicated to provide unique products and services that are second to none. Providing the best value to our customer will be a prime objective, and we recognize lowest cost does not always represent the best value.

Linkage to FAA Strategic Plan

FAA Strategic Goals, Key Initiatives, and Performance Goals

- The FAA has three key mission goals:

  - Safety—By 2007 reduce aviation fatal accident rates by 80 percent from 1996 levels.

  - Security—Prevent security incidents in the aviation system.

  - System Efficiency—Provide an aerospace transportation system that meets the needs of users and is efficient in the application of FAA and aerospace resources.

The FAALC in some way will contribute to the accomplishment of all of these goals; however, our mission is most directly related to the System Efficiency goal. The clear connection between our mission and this goal is illustrated in the FAA FY-2000 President's Budget Submission and Performance Plan. In that submission, the Agency's funding is linked to one of the three agency strategic goals. The source of our primary FAA customers' funding is tied directly to the System Efficiency goal. As a result, FAALC strategic goals and performance targets are aimed at improving the utilization of resources and achieving results that will improve operational availability of the NAS.

Strengths Weaknesses Opportunities and Threats Analysis Summary

FAALC strategies were developed based on a situational analysis considering current environmental factors, both internal and external, that could affect the future of the FAALC. The strengths, weaknesses, opportunities, and threats (SWOT) associated with each were also analyzed. The results of this SWOT analysis formed the basis for identification of our strategic objectives. We established objectives that leverage our strengths, eliminate our weaknesses, neutralize threats, and take advantage of opportunities.

A detailed discussion of the critical strengths, weaknesses, opportunities, and threats is provided in the Supplemental Strategic Guidance document.

Strategic Objectives, Measures and Targets

The FAALC Strategic objectives, measures, and targets were developed using the "Balanced Scorecard Approach." The Balanced Scorecard Approach says the success of an organization is dependent upon balancing various aspects of the organization to achieve overall success. Managers must look at the organization from four basic perspectives:

- **The Customer Perspective**—What must we do to satisfy and retain current customers and attract new customers? Customers in this context are primarily the end user of our products or services.

- **The Financial Stakeholder Perspective**—What must we do to satisfy our financial stakeholders? Our key financial stakeholders are the individuals and organizations that control or influence the appropriation, allocation, or utilization of Federal funds. Under the current financial management system, our financial stakeholders typically are not the end user of our products and services.

- **The Internal Business Perspective**—What core internal business processes drive the results we want to achieve under the customer perspective and the financial stakeholder perspective? For these processes, what level of performance must we achieve?

- **The Learning and Innovation Perspective**—What must we do to develop people and technology to support our internal business processes and improve our capabilities so that we can continue to add value to our cusotmers and our financial stakeholders?

The FAALC Balanced Scorecard consists of the following:

Strategies objectives translate our broad strategies into actionable goals in order to achieve our vision of the future.

Measures describe what we will measure to determine whether or not we have met our goals.

Targets for the measures are set 1 to 3 years out and are designed to s-t-r-e-t-c-h our performance.

The Customer Perspective

STRATEGIC OBJECTIVE	MEASURE	TARGET
● Increase customer satisfaction.	● Customer Satisfaction Rating.	● Close 15% of the gap between the April 1999 baseline of 3.66 and maximum rating of 5.0 for each 18-month rating cycle through 2002.
● Increase product availability for our customers.	● Customer Satisfaction Rating.	● Close 50% of the gap between the April 1999 baseline of 4.1 and importance to the customer rating of 4.5 for each 18-month rating cycle through 2002.
● Increase quality of items delivered.	● % Defective shipments (product defective). ● Customer survey rating for technical reliability. ● % Defective shipments (quantity, packing, packaging, marking, or wrong item basis for defective shipment). ● Customer survey rating for delivery accuracy.	● 50% decrease in reported defective products by 2002 based on FY99 defects per 1,000 issues. ● Close 33% of the gap between April 1999 baseline of 3.9 and importance rating of 4.5 for each 18-month rating cycle through 2002. ● 50% decrease in reported defective products by 2002 based on FY99 defects per 1,000 issues. ● Close 33% of the gap between the April 1999 baseline of 4.3 and importance rating of 4.6 for each 18-month rating cycle through 2002.
● Viewed by Agency as best value Logistics Support provider for life cycle support.	● Gross sales attributable to new systems workload.	● 5% increase in gross sales is attributable to new systems workload by 2002.

The Financial Stakeholder Perspective

STRATEGIC OBJECTIVE	MEASURE	TARGET
● Reduce cost.	● Repair cost.	● Reduce repair cost 10% over FY-99 baseline by 2002.
	● Inventory (stock) turn-over rate.	● Stock turnover rate improves by 10% each year through 2002.
	● PC&B as a ratio to gross margin.	● PC&B is 25% of gross margin by 2002.
	● Distribution cost per issue.	● 3% reduction in distribution cost per issue from baseline of $51.77 per issue by end of FY-2000.
● Achieve a return on investment for the Agency when selected to provide Logistics Support for new systems.	● Return on Investment (ROI) to Agency.	● ROI of at least 10% on new business.
● Increase gross sales.	● Volume of sales for products, services, and consulting.	● Increase gross sales 25% by 2002 using FY99 as a baseline.

The Internal Business Perspective

STRATEGIC OBJECTIVE	MEASURE	TARGET
• Reduce average repair time for LRU repair.	• Average repair time.	• Reduce average repair time for LRU in repair facilities 10% by FY-2002 over FY-99 baseline.
• Improve product delivery processes and systems.	• Number of customer orders filled in 24 hours.	• Increase number of customer orders filled in 24 hours by 50%. Include orders filled from FAALC Distribution Center stock only, not PDS shipments.
	• Customer returns receipted to stock within 24 hours.	• 100% of customer returns receipted to stock within 24 hours by 2002.
	• Inventory accuracy for quantity and location.	• 99% inventory accuracy by 2002.
	• Warehouse refusal rate.	• .1% refusal rate by 2002.
• Improve product innovation and technology insertion.	• ROI on obsolescence driven replacements at form, fit, and function.	• ROI greater than 10% per project.
• Improve internal cost analysis process and capabilities.	• Availability of valid financial information necessary to achieve financial objectives and targets related to cost reduction.	• Cost reduction goals under financial perspective are met. (Note: If goals are not met, the inability to meet the goals cannot be attributed to lack of valid financial reports or analyses.)

The Learning and Innovation Perspective

STRATEGIC OBJECTIVE	MEASURE	TARGET
Develop, train, and retain current workers. Attract, develop, and retain knowledge workers. Skills necessary to ensure product/service delivery are available.	Percentage of current competency inventories completed and training/development completed.	All occupations have a current competency inventory reflecting new competencies needed to meet future demands, and training matrix by end of FY 2000. All employees have completed identified training or development within 1 year after assuming current position or receiving new training matrix, providing funding for training is available.
Implement total asset tracking system, to include bar coding and other state of the art technology.	Implementation of total asset tracking system. (This measure tied to inventory accuracy, and other process measures in internal business perspective.)	Total asset tracking system implemented by end of FY-2000, and system produces real time asset location and movement information.
Implement effective internal cost accounting and financial management information system.	Availability of current cost information. Feedback from users.	100% of managers and supervisors have cost data available to them through an automated system by end of FY-2000. 100% of managers and supervisors indicate automated system is a useful tool for making operational decisions.
Encourage and facilitate self-development of managers.	Managerial 360 degree assessment.	Assessment indicates composite scores for all managers improved by .75 points over 1999 assessment by 2002. (Composite score is special report that summarizes scores for all managers into one value for the management team. Individual scores are not identifiable.)
All employees (including supervisory and non supervisory) are motivated and job satisfaction is high.	Employee attitude survey results.	FAALC results show an increase of at least .3 points in all measured categories for all employees over EAS conducted in 1998.
Implement effective shop production control system.	Production control efficiency index.	System is implemented and 100% of identified requirements in the index are rated satisfactory or higher by end of FY-2000.

Strategic Plan Deployment and Action Plans

Each Division and Group will develop annual business plans to describe how their organization will contribute to the achievement of the Strategic Objectives. Preparation of business plans is contingent upon having adequate cost and performance data to make projections and establish measurable goals and targets.

At a minimum business plans will include:

- Financial projections based on projected cost of operations, investments, and revenue.

- Resource utilization plan.

- Production plan indicating anticipated changes in existing workload, and any new workload the Division may be planning to assume or pursue with appropriate business case justification.

- Annual Division or Group goals. These goals must be tied to FAALC strategic objectives or FAALC annual goals.

- Results based performance measures and targets for each annual division goal.

- Outline of key milestones for any projects associated with FAALC strategic goals.

- Explanation regarding how Division or Group annual goals will be cascaded through all levels of the organization.

CHAPTER 4

The Balanced Scorecard at the Naval Undersea Warfare Center

The subject of the first case study is the Naval Undersea Warfare Center (NUWC) in Newport, Rhode Island, and Newport Division, a subordinate command. They have been using planning as a key business process for almost 20 years. Since 1981, Newport Division has used a 5-year planning process as the cornerstone of its management process.

NUWC's 1998 strategic plan is presented in its entirety in the pages that follow. The plan, which ends with a discussion of "Balanced Performance Measures," is one of the earliest examples of the use of this concept in a federal organization. Starting with this strategic plan, NUWC began assessing progress toward its strategic goals by looking at five perspectives: (1) customer perspective, (2) business perspective, (3) financial perspective, (4) employee perspective, and (5) learning and growth perspective. These performance measures are then reflected in 5-year plans throughout the divisions. On a quarterly basis, the commander and executive director review the performance of the organization on the basis of these five Balanced Performance Measures (BPMs).

The plan is followed by Figure 4–3, which illustrates NUWC strategic management. It is followed by the 1998 strategic plan for the Newport Division of NUWC. The plan, which is dated October 1, 1997, has a detailed section on BPMs.

Following the Newport Division strategic plan is the text of a three-fold handout explaining the major portions of the strategic plan and highlighting the five BPMs. Every large federal organization should publish a similar handout and send it to their employees. Its brevity will encourage workers to learn more about the strategic management process and heighten their interest in it.

The chapter continues with Figure 4–4, which illustrates the Fiscal Year (FY) 2001–2005 5-year planning process at NUWC, Newport Division. It is followed by the 5-year planning schedule (Figure 4–5) and the 5-year planning plan of action and milestones (Figure 4–6).

The chapter concludes with a March 2000 article from the NUWC newspaper. It explains the 5-year planning history and the relation of performance measurement and the Balanced Scorecard to this process.

NAVAL UNDERSEA WARFARE CENTER 1998 STRATEGIC PLAN

The following material is adapted from the Naval Undersea Warfare Center, *The NUWC Strategic Plan*, Newport, Rhode Island, NUWC, 1997.

Commander and Technical Director Message

We are witnessing a new era in national security where the phrase "Post-Cold War" is losing its relevance. The promise of technology and the Revolution in Military Affairs (and the accompanying Revolution in Business Affairs) have brought us to the threshold of a new era, one where we have unprecedented opportunity to forge our future. Since the previous version of our Strategic Plan was published in January 1996, we have seen significant changes in DoD and Navy policy guidance and considerable progress in government reinvention and acquisition reform. These changes and the unfolding challenges of the future have precipitated a renewed assessment of our strategic planning processes and led us to publish this document, our 1998 Strategic Plan.

In our previous plan, we discussed the challenges associated with the shift in Undersea Warfare emphasis from open ocean to the littoral and emphasized our responsibilities to lower our costs to the taxpayer while implementing cutting-edge Undersea Warfare technologies. These imperatives remain and have been underscored in new military strategy documents, including *Joint Vision 2010* and *Forward . . . from the Sea.* Our joint warfighting role is integral to the concepts in these and other documents, and our contributions to Joint Warfighting Capability Objectives are continually expanding. Our broadening responsibilities and the constrained funding environment demand our vigilance in accomplishing every aspect of our mission.

The Naval Undersea Warfare Center, its Divisions, and its components are well situated to meet the complex challenges ahead. We have the right mix of highly trained and motivated employees, state-of-the-art facilities and world-class processes to sustain our reputation for excellence that has been cultivated since our beginnings. Our record of accomplishment in support of the Naval Sea Systems Command and the end-users of our products in the Fleet stand as a tribute to the people who make up our workforce. As the pressures to provide more affordable and technologically effective products and services continue apace, we will rise to the challenge, using innovative approaches and learning from the successes of others. Keeping pace with the rapid advances in a broad array of technologies and processes, we will play a vital role in preserving our Navy's Undersea Warfare superiority well into the next millennium.

This Strategic Plan provides a conceptual framework for success in the 21st century. It requires the support of every NUWC employee to be effective. As a team that is focused on the future, we can provide the utmost support to NAVSEA, and more importantly, to the men and women of the finest Navy in the world.

RADM John F. Shipway
Commander

Dr. John E. Sirmalis
Technical Director

Introduction

The Naval Undersea Warfare Center (NUWC) is the Navy's full-spectrum research, development, test & evaluation (RDT&E), engineering, and fleet support center for submarines, autonomous underwater systems, and offensive and defensive weapons systems associated with Undersea Warfare. Having refined the roles of our two Divisions in supporting the operating forces of the Navy over the past five years, we are positioned to improve and expand our contributions in Undersea Warfare. We are revising our planning approach and our processes to provide high quality, affordable RDT&E, in-service engineering, and total life cycle support for the Navy's Undersea Warfare systems and capabilities.

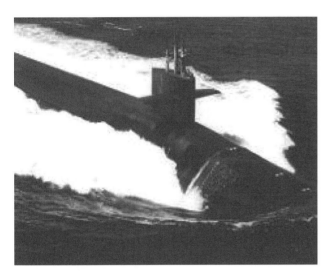

We must break down internal and external barriers to productivity and better understand our individual and collective roles in meeting the challenges ahead.

The NUWC Divisions today are lean, efficient, and focused on our customers' needs. We have evolved to adapt to diminishing resources and a diverse, diffused set of military threats; emphasized technologies that enable the Navy's Undersea Warfare operating forces to make better contributions in joint campaigns; and have established a position of leadership in government reinvention and acquisition reform. Nonetheless, the uncertainties ahead demand that we redouble our efforts to provide effective and affordable products and services to our customers. In the absence of a single, highly capable and well-defined threat, we must establish a flexible technological vision to drive our Undersea Warfare capabilities in the future. With technology and innovation as our primary tools, we have the opportunity to develop processes, products, and services that will further enhance the value of the Navy's Undersea Warfare capabilities. To achieve the necessary progress, we will have to look beyond our own organizations for good ideas and best practices from industry and academia, and to forge mutually beneficial cooperative alliances with other organizations. We must break down internal and external barriers to productivity and better understand our individual and collective roles in meeting the challenges ahead.

As the challenges of the future unfold, we must assess our progress toward our vision and goals and adjust our strategic plans accordingly. Therefore, we have revised our Strategic Plan to incorporate a new set of goals and action strategies to attain them. Our Strategic Plan complements national military strategy, the precepts of the National Performance Review (NPR), and the eight strategic goals outlined in NAVSEA's strategic plan. We fully embrace these strategic goals and will continue to integrate them into all aspects of internal planning. The NUWC Senior Management Team—consisting of the NUWC Commander and Technical Director; and the Division Commanders and Executive Directors—routinely meets to review NUWC's Strategic Plan, its implementation, and its effectiveness. These reviews have reinforced the validity of our planning and have served as a forum to develop objective measures of effectiveness.

Balanced Performance Measures

An important feature of our Strategic Plan is the establishment of a set of balanced performance measurements that allow[s] us to assess our progress toward achieving our strategic goals. Our performance will be appraised in five key perspectives: our customer perspective, our employee perspective, our internal business perspective, our financial perspective, and our learning and growth perspective. Within each of these areas, we have developed a list of more specific factors or requirements that provide standards against which we can better determine our progress. By integrating the performance measurements obtained in each of the five perspectives, we can adjust our processes or plans as necessary to stay on the appropriate path to the future.

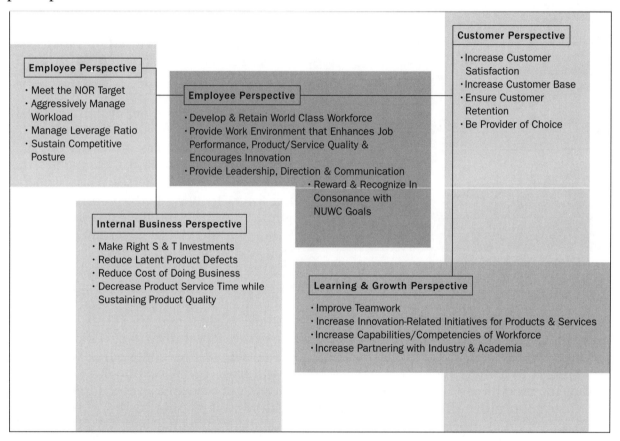

Strategic Overview

The NUWC Strategic Plan is published for our employees and stakeholders to keep them informed of our general direction and guidance. It details our vision for the future and the strategic goals we have set to attain that vision. It is intended to focus our collective efforts on a common approach to meet future challenges and it defines our corporate philosophy.

The five strategic goals contained in this document are aligned with NAVSEA's strategic goals and support the spirit and intent of the Government Performance and Results Act (GPRA) and the National Partnership for Reinventing Government (NPR) by directing the establishment of measures that improve performance and reduce costs. Additionally, this plan's Operating Principles are related to and supportive of NAVSEA's Guiding Principles.

Our Strategic Plan is the cornerstone of our strategic planning process. In response to a broad array of external factors, including military strategy, funding constraints, and, most importantly, the Navy's warfighting requirements, we must routinely evaluate our strategic approach and adjust our plans and processes to most effectively accomplish our mission. Based upon DoD, Navy, and NAVSEA guidance and anticipated resources, our plan assesses how best to accomplish our mission and achieve our vision. Our strategic goals and their associated action strategies were developed with the needs and expectations of our customers as primary considerations. Our plan also incorporates a key aspect of the GPRA by addressing performance measurement. By using a Balanced Scorecard approach, we will have defined performance metrics that help us assess our progress toward attaining each goal.

The NUWC Strategic Plan plays a fundamental role in our strategic planning processes. Figure 4–1 illustrates the overall strategic planning process, and demonstrates how the cycle is influenced continually by obtaining feedback and adjusting our processes or plans accordingly.

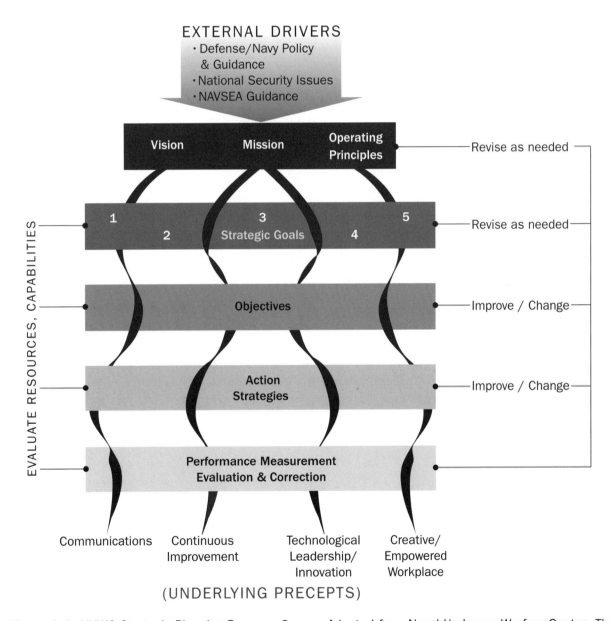

Figure 4–1. NUWC Strategic Planning Process. *Source:* Adapted from Naval Undersea Warfare Center, *The NUWC Strategic Plan,* Newport, Rhode Island, NUWC, 1997.

Vision/Mission/Charter Leadership Areas

Vision

Be our Nation's provider of choice for Undersea Superiority, satisfying today's needs and meeting tomorrow's challenges.

Mission—Undersea Superiority: Today and Tomorrow

We provide the technical foundation, which enables the conceptualization, research, development, fielding, modernization, in-service engineering, and maintenance of systems that ensure our Navy's undersea superiority.

Corporate Charter

The NUWC Charter, promulgated in December 1992, established the top-level organizational relationships (Figure 4–2) and technical leadership areas for NUWC and expertise in the following technical areas:

Technical leadership areas

As assigned by SECNAVINST 5400.16 of 18 December 1992, NUWC provides the Navy with leadership in:

- Undersea Warfare Modeling and Analysis
- Submarine Combat and Combat Control Systems
- Surface Ship and Submarine Sonar Systems
- Submarine Electronic Warfare
- Submarine Unique On-Board Communications Systems and Communications Nodes
- Submarine Launched Weapons Systems (except Strategic Ballistic Missile Systems, Cruise Missiles, and Related Systems)
- Undersea Ranges
- Torpedoes and Torpedo Countermeasures
- Submarine Vulnerability and Survivability (except Hull, Mechanical & Electrical Ship's Equipment—HM&E)
- Undersea Vehicle Active and Passive Signatures (except HM&E)
- Submarine Electromagnetic, Electro-optic and Nonacoustic-effects Reconnaissance, Search and Track Systems

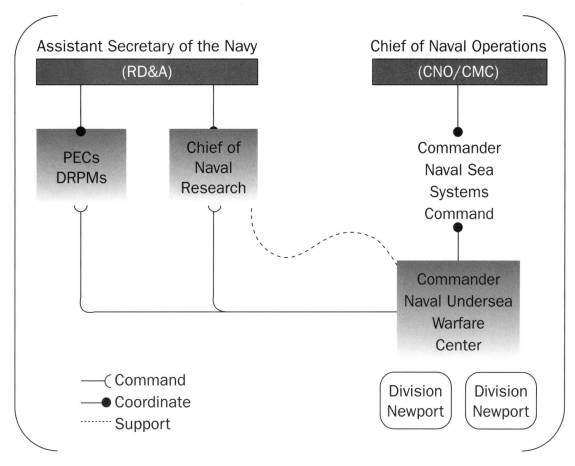

Figure 4–2. Naval Undersea Warfare Center Organizational Structure & Operating Relationships. *Source:* Adapted from Naval Undersea Warfare Center, *The NUWC Strategic Plan,* Newport, Rhode Island, NUWC, 1997.

Operating Principles

Our Operating Principles provide a foundation that governs our approach to daily operations. They are interrelated by several underlying precepts that should influence everything we do:

- Open communications, internally and externally;
- Continuous improvement;
- Technological leadership and innovation; and
- A creative, empowered workforce.

NUWC's operating principles are:

Our customers come first. Understanding and responding to their current and emerging needs are our top priorities. We will collaborate closely with our customers and other stakeholders to ensure we meet their requirements for performance, affordability, and timeliness.

Our employees are the key to our success. Our employees are our most valuable resource. We will provide them with a productive work environment and the necessary skill set, knowledge, and incentives to accomplish our mission.

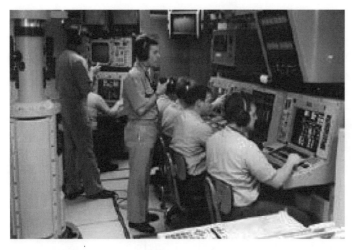

We are committed to continuous improvement of products, processes, and services. Using the best management practices, we will make improvement decisions based on fact and knowledge. We will measure our performance and, using benchmarking, continuously evaluate our progress toward our goals.

Teamwork is essential. We work as dedicated and effective partners with our family of customers, suppliers, and stakeholders. We will share and pursue the NUWC vision as a unified team.

Innovation and creativity are critical to our success. We seek new and imaginative approaches in creating technologically advanced products and in developing effective business processes to meet our customers' current and future needs.

We value diversity. We recognize and respect the benefits of diversity and are committed to recruiting and developing a diverse workforce.

Environmental stewardship and safety are crucial. Our practices will foster a safe work environment for our employees, provide safe and environmentally sound products for our customers, and ensure we are prudent stewards of the environment.

We conduct ourselves in an ethical manner. We are accountable to the American public and are committed to the highest ethical standards.

Strategic Goals, Objectives, and Strategies

This plan provides a blueprint that charts how we will make our vision a reality. The five goals presented below establish the direction we will take in accomplishing our mission and fulfilling our obligations to the Navy, DoD, and the taxpayer over the next several years. Each goal is supported by more specific objectives and strategies, which help to further refine how we will satisfy current and future undersea superiority requirements. The objectives represent "what" NUWC intends to accomplish with respect to its overarching strategic goal, and the strategies indicate "how" we will achieve each goal. Pursuing these objectives and strategies will allow us to use the appropriate combination of best practices, in both our business and technical processes, and team spirit to enable our delivery of products and services that are effective, affordable, and timely.

Strategic Goal 1

Customer satisfaction

Objectives:

- Refine our ability to anticipate customer needs and expectations.
- Maintain an open, frank relationship with customers to enhance our responsiveness.
- Work closely with our customers to determine their needs.

Strategies:

- Enhance cooperative alliances with customers, sponsors, and suppliers to improve communication of expectations and needs and to encourage increased participation among stakeholders.

- Assign NUWC personnel where appropriate to improve customer satisfaction.
- Develop methods to systematically survey customer satisfaction in our performance as well as their anticipated needs and concerns.
- Foster a spirit of dedication to customers throughout NUWC.

Strategic Goal 2

Enhance the effectiveness of the NUWC workforce by providing opportunity for all employees to realize their full potential

Objectives:

- Develop the tools to ensure a well-informed, skilled, and innovative workforce that is empowered and best equipped to seek new opportunities while accommodating change.
- Expand cross-training, improve internal communications, and promote sharing of ideas throughout NUWC.
- Provide a work environment that enhances productivity, safety, and quality of life.

Strategies:

- Refine human resources plans to achieve a flexible organization based on anticipated work requirements and critical technical capabilities and supporting skills.
- Provide for the professional development of a diverse and highly capable, right-sized workforce.
- Pursue innovative human resources policies to improve productivity through Reinvention Laboratory and Personnel Demonstration programs.
- Recognize and reward employee achievements.
- Encourage employee participation in decision processes that shape the future of the workforce and the organization.
- Detect and break down barriers to communications.

Strategic Goal 3

Improve the responsiveness, performance, and efficiency of NUWC in the conduct of all processes

Objectives:

- Implement process improvements and better business practices.
- Develop and implement cutting-edge acquisition reform and government reinvention measures.
- Improve our ability to provide decisive and prompt action in responding to short-fused requirements.

Strategies:

- Identify technical and business process improvements to achieve better performance, effectiveness, and efficiency.
- Explore internal and external sources for best practices, and implement those that will improve NUWC's performance.
- Eliminate redundant and non-value-added practices.
- Encourage sharing of ideas and lessons learned by promoting strong intra- and inter-divisional reliance programs.
- Pursue technologies that affordably enhance processes and business practices and add product and service value to the customer.

Strategic Goal 4

Develop affordable products and services that fully address Navy needs and lower total ownership costs

Objectives:

- Maintain leadership in enabling the development and maintenance of technologically superior, affordable, and effective products and services.
- Sustain the capability to rapidly and affordably upgrade or correct problems in existing fleet systems.
- Provide best value products and services that meet customers' needs.
- Improve maintenance capabilities and lower costs by improving work practices.
- Sustain capability to meet emergent customer requirements.

Strategies:

- Implement innovative processes that will eliminate inefficiencies and will improve overall cost effectiveness.
- Consider total ownership costs as a primary factor in all acquisition endeavors.
- Use applicable commercial practices and technologies and enhance our knowledge of best practices by capitalizing upon collaborative alliances with industry and academia.
- Strive to lower total life cycle costs without sacrificing warfighting capabilities.
- Encourage increased communications and collaborations across the Divisions to cultivate and share relevant undersea warfare technologies and best practices.
- Work with customers to explore alternative methods to address their needs and resource constraints.

Strategic Goal 5

Apply innovative approaches to meet future challenges

Objectives:

- Aggressively seek and deploy innovative new technologies, which will sustain the Navy's Undersea Warfare competitive advantage.
- Eliminate technical insularity and promote free exchange of ideas.
- Build on successful innovative approaches used by other organizations.
- Provide affordable, high-quality technical, support, and industrial facilities that are unique and essential to Submarine and Undersea Warfare.
- Develop advanced concepts in Undersea Warfare to meet future needs.

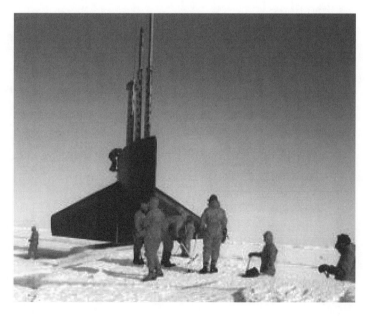

Strategies:

- Anticipate undersea superiority emerging needs and their potential implications.

- Consider current and projected customer needs in assessing innovative technologies or processes.
- Pursue advanced concepts that will lead to breakthrough technologies.
- Develop processes to quickly deploy new technologies that accelerate development cycles, improve performance, and lower costs.
- Expand our knowledge base in Undersea Warfare and joint warfighting mission areas.
- Pursue cooperative alliances with industry, academia, other government agencies, and allies to identify and capture technology insertion opportunities.
- Ensure our key technical and support facilities are appropriately used, refined, and revitalized to meet current and future requirements.

NUSC STRATEGIC MANAGEMENT PROCESS

Figure 4–3 depicts the NUWC strategic management process.

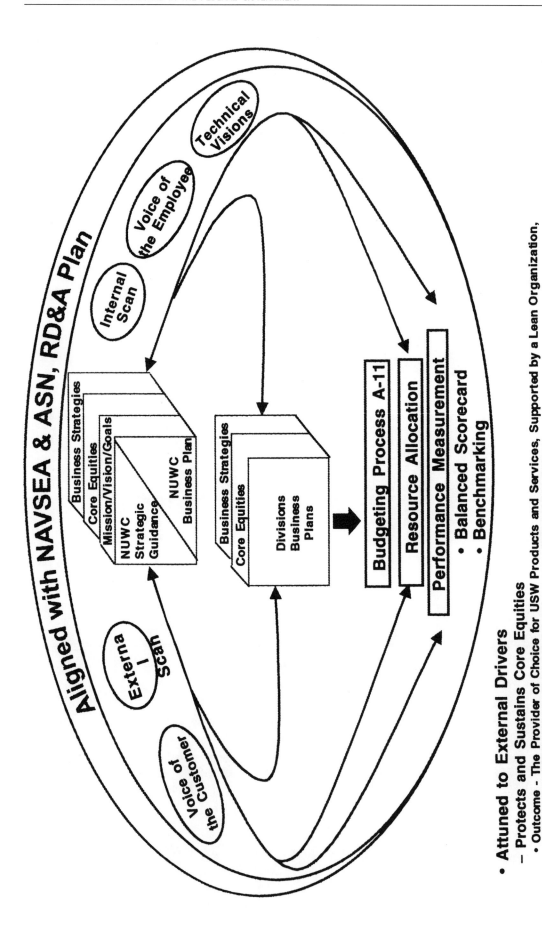

Figure 4–3. NUWC Strategic Management Process. *Source:* Head, Strategy Development Staff (Code 011), Naval Undersea Warfare Center, Division Newport, Newport, Rhode Island.

NUWC NEWPORT DIVISION 1998 STRATEGIC PLAN

The following material is adapted from *Strategic Plan 1998: Naval Undersea Warfare Center Division Newport,* Newport, Rhode Island, Naval Undersea Warfare Center Division Newport, 1997, Report No. NUWC-NPT-AP10,852-1.

STRATEGIC
PLAN

1998

we enable undersea superiority,

SATISFYING TODAY'S *needs*

and meeting tomorrow's CHALLENGES...

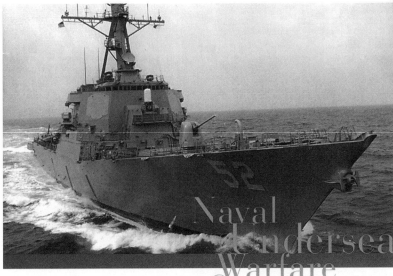

Naval
Undersea
Warfare
Center
Division Newport

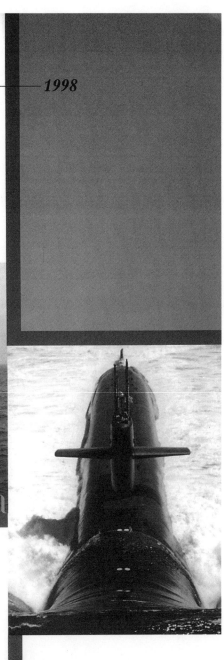

COMMANDER AND EXECUTIVE DIRECTOR MESSAGE

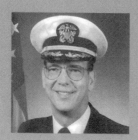

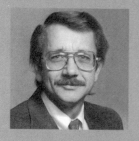

The dedication and resourcefulness of our workforce has resulted in a rich legacy of achievement in effective undersea warfare products and services. As a result, we have a great heritage in which we can take great pride and satisfaction. However, tremendous changes have occurred in the past five years since we formed the Naval Undersea Warfare Center, and new changes continue at an increasingly intense pace. In this demanding environment we cannot let our proud past distract us from addressing the challenges of change. We must continue our tradition of excellence, but we must also adapt so we can sustain it in a much different world. This strategic plan provides a framework for building our future. It describes the strategic foundation and our strategic management processes that are built upon it; explains our strategic goals, what they mean to us, and how we will attain them; and it relates the plan to our five-year planning process and the balanced performance measures system for evaluating our progress.

Our future is one of continued changes, constraints, and heightened competition for increasingly scarce national security resources. We must fully understand and satisfy our customers' needs of today while anticipating and preparing for future needs. Our technical and business practices must be fine-tuned so we can provide capable and affordable products and services more quickly. Continued rapid advances in technology throughout the marketplace challenge us to forge new relationships with others and to build new competencies and learn new skills.

When faced with the challenges of the future, we should frame our actions in the form of four underlying precepts: we should communicate with whomever appropriate to exchange knowledge and ideas; we must remember that each of us has leadership and accountability responsibilities that we cannot ignore; we should strive for innovation and new ideas to help us work smarter, faster, and more affordably; and we must establish productive collaborations that optimize use of scarce resources and maximize product quality.

Our greatest strength continues to be you, our employees. This plan provides a conceptual blueprint for our evolution, and the key to its success lies in each of you. We ask that you read and embrace this plan. If we are to continue to be successful, each of you must take a proactive role in crafting the solutions to the challenges and changes that we face. Our success demands that each of you assume an active role in forging our future. We look forward to working with you in our journey of change and, as always, welcome your ideas and feedback.

S. J. LOGUE
CAPTAIN, U.S. NAVY
COMMANDER

J. G. KEIL
EXECUTIVE DIRECTOR

TABLE OF CONTENTS

Strategic **Framework**   2

Cultural Values/Operating Principles   4

Strategic GOALS   6
   Increase Customer Loyalty
   Invest in Our People
   Improve the Way We Work
   Provide Capable and Affordable Products
   Innovate for the Future

BALANCED **Performance** *Measures*   12

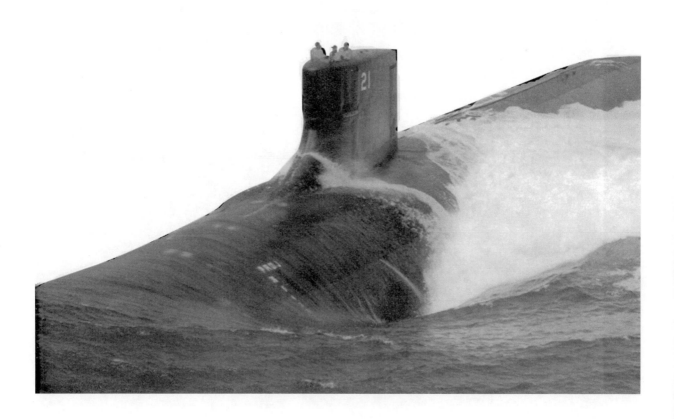

STRATEGIC FRAMEWORK

Our Mission

UNDERSEA SUPERIORITY: TODAY AND TOMORROW.

We provide the technical foundation that enables the conceptualization, research, development, fielding, modernization, and maintenance of systems that ensure our Navy's undersea superiority.

Our Vision

Be our Nation's provider of choice for undersea superiority, satisfying today's needs and meeting tomorrow's challenges.

OUR MISSION IS OUR REASON FOR BEING... *our responsibility for fulfilling the Navy's and the Nation's defense needs.* Our Vision represents the future state we strive to achieve in accomplishing our mission. In working toward our vision, we consider a number of external and internal factors: we conduct a continuous External Scan to determine what conditions or actions are currently influencing

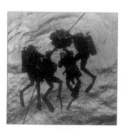 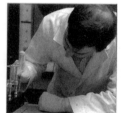

or will influence our ability to meet our mission, including policy, resources, competitors, and developments in industry; Customer Feedback gives us important information regarding our customers' view of our performance and provides insight into means for improving; and Employee Feedback conveys our employees' perspective on how we can improve ourselves. These factors shape and drive our approach to the future, and our actions are "filtered" through our system of Cultural Values and our Operating Principles (see following pages). This process results in establishment of our STRATEGIC GOALS, which when attained will permit us to *achieve our vision and accomplish* We develop strategies for meeting each Strategic Goal and use a balanced set of performance measures to continually assess our progress toward goal attainment.

2

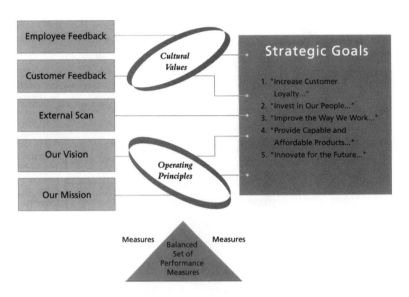

In implementing our action strategies, we will continually measure our progress through systematic assessments of performance against goals and their support-

ing operating targets. This allows us to make adjustments to our management processes to ensure we are headed toward the goal. The strategies that we refine and pursue at the Division Newport level serve as the basis for the five-year plans that are developed and deployed throughout our departments.

Our strategic management process is supportive of the strategic plans and the mission attainment of both the Naval Sea Systems Command (NAVSEA) and the Naval Undersea Warfare Center (NUWC). This "co-missioning" ensures that our efforts are aligned with and fully support NAVSEA and NUWC strategic goals.

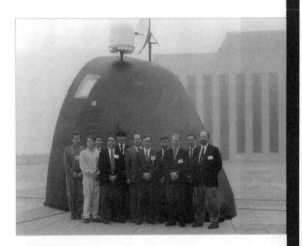

our mission.   In the following pages, we explain our cultural values, operating principles, and strategic goals. Each of our strategic goals and the strategies we will use to achieve them are explained in terms of both our employees' perspective and Division management's perspective.

3

OUR CULTURAL VALUES

Our cultural values influence everything we do; they make up our fundamental system of beliefs, which describe how we approach our responsibilities.

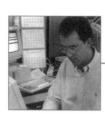
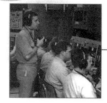

"Our Commitment is to
Our CUSTOMERS*"*

Team Members
Sponsors
Fleet
Citizens

"Our Strength is in
Our PEOPLE*"*

Responsive
Creative
Open
Empowered

"Our Contribution is in
Our PRODUCTS*"*

Innovative
Timely
Capable
Affordable

OUR OPERATING PRINCIPLES

Our operating principles reinforce and refine our cultural values, describing in more detail our "corporate philosophy." They are meant to serve as general guidelines for how we conduct our day-to-day business, and they provide a philosophical linkage between the way we carry out our routine activities and achieve our strategic goals. The following are our operating principles:

Our CUSTOMERS *come first.*

Working with our customers, we respond to the needs of the Fleet to ensure we provide the most effective and affordable undersea warfare products and services in a timely manner.

Our WORKFORCE *is critical to our success.*

We provide our workforce with the skill set, knowledge, motivation, and work environment to effectively accomplish our mission. We rely on our workforce to forge the future of the Division.

4

DIVERSITY *strengthens our creativity and teamwork.* We respect each other and our differences and recognize the value of our diverse backgrounds.

IMPROVEMENT *must be continuous.* We have a passion for excellence! We understand and support quality programs, and constantly work to enhance our processes, products, and services.

TEAMWORK *is essential.* We cooperate, communicate, and collaborate, both internally and externally, to achieve the most effective products and services.

INNOVATION *and creativity are crucial.* We seek new and innovative approaches to old problems and attack new challenges with imagination. We look outward for creative ideas to adapt to our use. We take manageable risks to field new technologies for effective solutions.

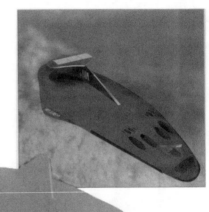

We are ACCOUNTABLE. We are honest, ethical, and accountable for all our actions.

We are COMMITTED *to environmental stewardship and safety.* We promote practices and attitudes that respect our environment and make our workplace safe and productive.

We are good CITIZENS *of our community.* We recognize our economic and social impact on the stakeholders in our communities. We adhere to the highest standards of citizenship and participate in charitable, educational, and community outreach programs.

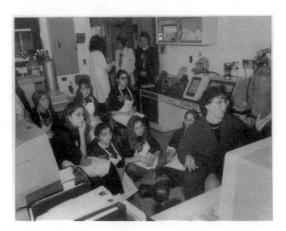

5

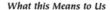

STRATEGIC GOAL 1

Increase Customer Loyalty ...

We will achieve this Goal by

- Fostering a spirit of dedication to customer satisfaction and service throughout Division Newport.

- Working closely with customers, maintaining frank and open relationships.

- Recognizing that each employee is an agent of the Division who carries our message to current and future customers.

- Initiating processes to improve customer loyalty and better address their concerns.

- Producing and providing best value products and services.

What this Means to Us

We must achieve and sustain high levels of customer loyalty if we expect to thrive as the Navy's primary provider of undersea warfare products and services. We can accomplish this only if we understand our customers' requirements and satisfy their needs. A second critical element of our strategy is to respond quickly to customer requests, questions, and comments. Additionally, we must constantly evaluate whether we are meeting customers' needs by asking them, through both formal survey processes and ongoing informal communications, how our performance compares with their expectations. Every one of us has the potential to positively (or negatively) impact customer loyalty. In all our customer interactions, we must be sensitive to and manage the image we project, both individually and collectively, to ensure it accurately portrays our capabilities and potential. This means

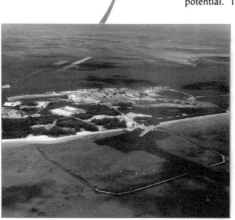

- Being honest, straightforward, and attentive with customers and sponsors.

- Seeking and sharing important information about customers that could impact our ability to meet their present and future needs.

- Keeping abreast of technological and warfighting issues that are important to our customers and stakeholders.

- Acting as positive representatives of the Division, keeping customers informed of our technical accomplishments, innovations, awards, and other relevant information that will increase their confidence in our products and services.

- Taking prompt action to address causes of customer concern or dissatisfaction.

- Creating opportunities to exceed customer expectations.

6 CUSTOMER *Loyalty*

Strategies

- Conduct periodic surveys of customers, analyzing and internally disseminating results; take prompt, decisive action to address customer concerns.

- Conduct open and frank discussions of expectations, concerns, ideas, and opportunities with customers and stakeholders; follow up with appropriate actions.

- Anticipate and position for emergent customer needs.

- Develop cooperative alliances with customers, sponsors, and suppliers to enhance customer satisfaction.

- Celebrate and share our successes with our customers.

- Assign personnel to field positions with customers.

Invest in Our People...

STRATEGIC GOAL 2

We will achieve this Goal by

- Providing challenging work and development opportunities to all members of our organization at every level.

- Establishing a work atmosphere that promotes loyalty, trust, cooperation, productivity, and innovation.

- Placing high priority on addressing employee challenges and concerns.

- Developing an agile, flexible, and effective workforce.

- Encouraging our people to become well-informed and innovative, to look beyond traditional boundaries for solutions, and to welcome the opportunities and challenges associated with the processes of continuous, adaptive, or breakthrough change.

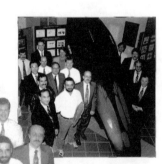

What this Means to Us

Employee knowledge, skill, and team spirit are essential to our success. Each of us must possess a strong and enduring desire to improve individual and organizational performance. Our workforce will be characterized as energetic, spirited, agile, proactive, and future-focused. This means

- Pursuing challenging opportunities to develop professional and managerial knowledge and skills.

- Mentoring fellow employees.

- Being familiar with and supporting Division management initiatives.

7

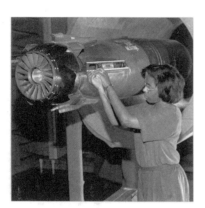

- Communicating openly, sharing information, and listening for understanding.

- Taking responsibility for job performance.

Strategies

- Enhance workforce professional development through training, challenging field assignments and educational programs, and by encouraging employee participation in development processes.

- Conduct employee surveys and use results to generate improvements.

- Keep each other well informed.

- Implement hiring and retention strategies that meet strategic skill set needs.

- Provide the necessary tools and facilities to enable workforce effectiveness.

- Pursue innovative human resources policies and plans.

- Foster among supervisors a heightened appreciation of the present and future challenges facing employees.

- Hold employees accountable for work performance, recognizing and rewarding individual and team contributions.

STRATEGIC GOAL 3

Improve the Way We Work...

We will achieve this Goal by

- Questioning what we do and why we do it.

- Making continuous improvements in technical and business processes.

- Measuring results and improving/adapting processes from measurement and facts.

- Streamlining or eliminating inefficient or wasteful processes/practices.

- Managing total ownership costs.

- Doing more with less and working better/cheaper/faster.

- Infusing cost-consciousness into all business decisions to balance technical positioning for the future.

What this Means to Us

This goal is important to every part of our organization, product lines as well as business departments. Each of us must improve our overall performance while reducing bottom-line costs to our customers. To succeed at this difficult task, each of us has to constantly re-examine how we approach every aspect of our

8

work. Although measures that enhance our effectiveness can be initiated from the top down, workers at local levels know best how to improve performance, and therefore we must be actively involved in helping achieve the National Performance Review goal of more effective operations. This means

- Examining local processes and practices continuously to determine if and how they might be improved, asking "How can I do my job better?" every day.

- Working as a team.

- Supporting Division-wide management initiatives introduced to increase effectiveness and/or reduce costs.

- Seeking and sharing good ideas/best practices that could be adopted across departmental lines.

- Communicating ideas up and down the chain of command, and across the Division.

Strategies

- Find, share, and implement new ideas and best practices from other organizations.

- Capitalize on government initiatives and reinvention laboratory status.

- Work closely with NUWC Division Keyport to draw from each other's strengths.

- Apply new organizational effectiveness concepts to make the Division more effective and efficient.

- Use cross- and intra-departmental reliance to capitalize on our strengths throughout the Division.

- Use performance measurement to assess cost-effectiveness and overall performance.

- Create incentives to eliminate wasteful, duplicative, and no-consequence work.

- Realize technical process improvements to enhance performance and achieve targeted cost/schedule reductions.

- Maintain competitive costs to customers.

- Establish and manage to appropriate business operating targets.

- Pursue technologies that enhance effectiveness.

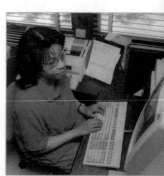

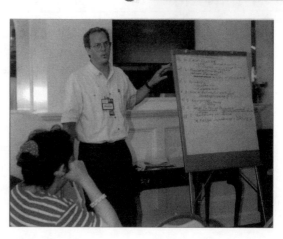

Continuous IMPROVEMENT

9

STRATEGIC GOAL 4

Provide Capable and Affordable Products...

We will achieve this Goal by

- Understanding thoroughly the Fleet's operating environment and requirements to ensure effective products and solutions.

- Seeking and adopting innovative processes that will improve overall performance, reliability, and affordability.

- Providing prompt and comprehensive responses to short-fused Fleet requests.

- Generating new ideas to complement our technical capabilities and improve cost-effectiveness.

What this Means to Us

The warfighters in the Fleet depend upon us to provide undersea warfare systems that ensure unchallenged naval supremacy. To accomplish this vital part of our mission with constrained resources, we must use the most effective and affordable technologies available, and must refine our system concepts and implementation approaches to ensure that the total ownership costs of our products are kept to an absolute minimum. This means

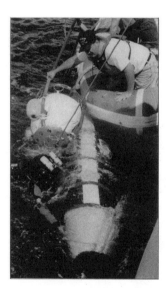

- Seizing opportunities to interact with our customers and the Fleet.

- Responding quickly and completely to customer requests.

- Developing "out of the box" solutions to the Navy's near-term challenges.

- Being creative, using and sharing ideas that lead to more effective and affordable products and services.

- Anticipating and meeting customer requirements, never losing sight of end-user needs.

- Capitalizing on commercial practices and technologies.

Strategies

- Support OPNAV and the Fleet in defining technical requirements.

- Exploit emergent technologies (e.g., simulation-based design, synthetic training environments, etc.) that enhance product quality.

- Improve communications with customers to quickly ascertain emergent Fleet requirements and to provide faster response.

- Devise and implement engineering practices and approaches that decrease cycle times and costs while enhancing product performance.

- Streamline or eliminate practices and processes that cause unnecessary delays in deployment or reduce effectiveness of our products.

10

- Pursue cross-departmental and external collaborations as a means to derive solutions that drive down costs and development times while improving product performance.

- Use a total systems engineering perspective in developing and applying technical processes.

Innovate for the Future...

**STRATEGIC
GOAL 5**

We will achieve this Goal by

- Engaging customers to understand and anticipate their future needs.

- Seeking the knowledge and mastery of technologies that will address long-term Fleet needs and sustain the Navy's competitive advantage in undersea warfare.

- Developing a global perspective and a corporate culture that foster innovation, eliminate technical insularity, and promote free exchange of ideas with our partners.

- Developing advanced concepts and processes to accelerate the transition of relevant, affordable new technologies to Fleet products.

- Ensuring our facilities and other resources are appropriately used, refined, and revitalized to support our customers' technology requirements.

What this Means to Us

The dynamic defense acquisition environment and rapidly advancing technology have brought us increasing opportunities for change. We are being provided with greater freedom and more tools with which we can address challenges and stretch our technical imagination. As we seek new and innovative options to expand the "art of the possible" in undersea warfare, we must channel our efforts into developing the right technologies and practices to achieve our technical visions. This means

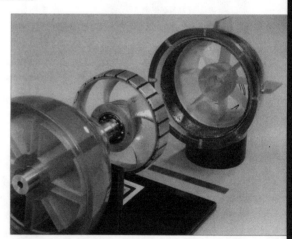

- Building broader and deeper understanding of current and expected undersea warfare military needs through education, professional development, and meaningful assignments.

- Broadening our technical horizons by increasing contacts with industry, academia, and other government agencies, and by looking beyond traditional bounds for ideas and information (i.e., developing a global perspective).

11

- Expanding the "art of the possible" by being creative and imaginative in developing technical visions for the future and identifying opportunities for technology insertion into current and future platforms and systems.

- Learning which tools and resources are available and applying them to address technological requirements.

Strategies
- Refine and apply warfare analysis methods and advanced concepts to better anticipate and assess military requirements.

- Create and deploy technical visions that drive and shape technology insertion opportunities.

- Collaborate with agencies and organizations that have strong potential to contribute to our technical knowledge.

- Pursue internal and external opportunities to leverage investments in technology.

- Encourage innovative technological approaches to undersea warfare challenges, allowing managed "risk-taking."

- Devise and utilize an employee development strategy that fosters the Division's growth as a learning organization.

- Develop a revitalization strategy for our facilities.

BALANCED PERFORMANCE MEASURES

Division Newport will assess its progress toward the strategic goals by using a set of balanced performance measurements. We have determined five key perspectives that serve as focal points for measuring our progress.

- Our customers' perspective, which examines how well we are meeting their needs.

- Our business perspective, where we examine our internal processes.

- Our financial perspective, or how we are managing our resources.

- Our employees' perspective, which will gauge adequacy of the work environment and whether we are giving employees the tools they need to meet expected demands.

- Our learning and growth perspective, where we examine our ability to learn and grow as an organization.

For each of these five interrelated perspectives, we have developed a list of performance criteria or goals that we intend to satisfy (see following page). At the Division level, these performance measures are deliberately broad to address strategic issues. As they are deployed throughout our product lines and business departments, they will provide a link between our high-level strategic goals and desired outcomes at the operational level. To serve their purpose, these performance measures, tailored to department needs, should be reflected in five-year plans throughout the Division.

12

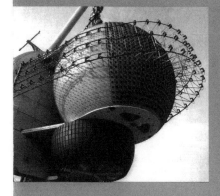

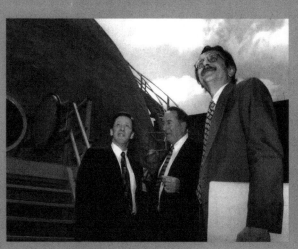

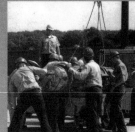

Measures

BALANCE

Internal Business Perspective

- Increase Science & Technology funding
- Increase advanced development funding
- Reduce cost of doing business
- Reduce latent Fleet defects
- Bring technical processes under process management
- Achieve seamless information flow

Customer Perspective

- Increase customer satisfaction
- Increase customer base
- Ensure customer retention
- Be provider of choice

Financial Perspective

- Meet the Net Operating Result target
- Sustain high efficiency
- Sustain/increase employee work base
- Manage leverage ratio

Learning and Growth Perspective

- Improve teamwork
- Increase innovation-related initiatives for product and services
- Increase capabilities/competencies of workforce
- Increase partnering with industry and academia

Employee Perspective

- Recruit, develop, and retain a world-class workforce
- Provide work environment that enhances job performance, product/ service quality, and encourages innovation
- Provide leadership, direction, and communication
- Reward and recognize in consonance with Division goals

NUWC NEWPORT DIVISION 1998 STRATEGIC PLAN BROCHURE

The material that follows is adapted from *Strategic Plan 1998: Naval Undersea Warfare Center Division Newport,* Newport, Rhode Island, Naval Undersea Warfare Center Division Newport, 1997, Report No. NUWC-NPT-AP10,852-2.

Mission

Undersea Superiority: Today and Tomorrow.
We provide the technical foundation that enables the conceptualization, research, development, fielding, modernization, and maintenance of systems that ensure our Navy's undersea superiority.

Vision

Be our Nation's provider of choice for undersea superiority, satisfying today's needs and meeting tomorrow's challenges.

Cultural Values

Our cultural values influence everything we do; they make up our fundamental system of beliefs, which describe how we approach our responsibilities.

"Our commitment is to our customers"

"Our strength is in our people"

"Our contribution is in our products"

Our Goals

Increase Customer Loyalty...

- Conduct periodic surveys of customers, analyzing and internally disseminating results; take prompt, decisive action to address customer concerns.
- Conduct open and frank discussions of expectations, concerns, ideas, and opportunities with customers and stakeholders; follow up with appropriate actions.
- Anticipate and position for emergent customer needs.
- Develop cooperative alliances with customers, sponsors, and suppliers to enhance customer satisfaction.
- Celebrate and share our successes with our customers.
- Assign personnel to field positions with customers.

Invest in Our People...

- Enhance workforce professional development through training, challenging field assignments and educational programs, and by enhancing employee participation in development processes.
- Conduct employee surveys and use results to generate improvements.
- Keep each other well-informed.
- Implement hiring and retention strategies that meet strategic skill set needs.
- Provide the necessary tools and facilities to enable workforce effectiveness.
- Pursue innovative human resources policies and plans.
- Foster among supervisors a heightened appreciation of the present and future challenges facing employees.
- Hold employees accountable for work performance, recognizing and rewarding individual and team contributions.

Improve the Way We Work...

- Find, share, and implement new ideas and best practices.
- Capitalize on government initiatives and reinvention laboratory status.
- Work closely with NUWC Division Keyport to draw from each other's strengths.
- Apply new organizational effectiveness concepts to make the Division more effective and efficient.
- Use cross- and intra-departmental reliance to capitalize on our strengths.
- Use performance measurement to assess cost-effectiveness and overall performance.
- Create incentives to eliminate wasteful or no-consequence work.
- Realize technical process improvements to enhance performance and achieve targeted cost/schedule reductions.
- Maintain competitive costs to customers.
- Establish and manage to appropriate business operating targets.
- Pursue technologies that enhance effectiveness.

Provide Capable and Affordable Products...

- Support OPNAV and the Fleet in defining technical requirements.
- Exploit emergent technologies (e.g., simulation-based design, synthetic training environments, etc.) that enhance product quality.
- Improve communications with customers to quickly ascertain emergent Fleet requirements and to provide faster response.
- Devise and implement engineering practices and approaches that decrease cycle times and costs while enhancing product performance.
- Streamline or eliminate practices and processes that cause unnecessary delays in deployment or reduce effectiveness of our products.
- Pursue cross-departmental and external collaborations as a means to derive solutions that drive down costs and development times while improving product performance.
- Use a total systems engineering perspective in technical processes.

Innovate for the Future...

- Refine and apply warfare analysis methods and advanced concepts to better anticipate and assess military requirements.
- Create and deploy technical visions that drive and shape technology insertion opportunities.
- Collaborate with agencies and organizations that have strong potential to contribute to our technical knowledge.
- Pursue opportunities to leverage investments in technology.
- Encourage innovative technological approaches to undersea warfare challenges, allowing managed "risk-taking".
- Devise and utilize an employee development strategy that fosters the Division's growth as a learning organization.
- Develop a revitalization strategy for our facilities.

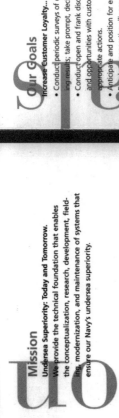

Balanced Performance Measures

- Customer Perspective
- Internal Business Perspective
- Learning and Growth Perspective
- Financial Perspective
- Employee Perspective

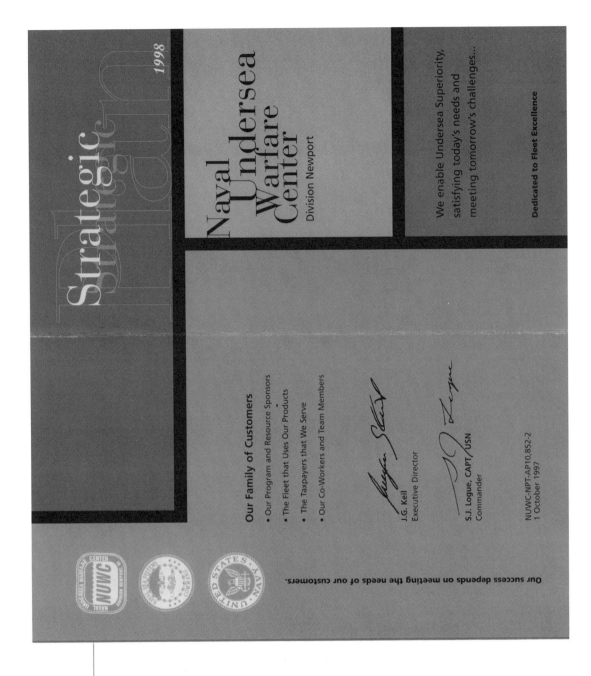

NUWC NEWPORT DIVISION 5-YEAR PLANNING PROCESS

Figure 4–4 depicts the FY01–05 5-year planning process, while Figure 4–5 presents the 5-year planning schedule. The 5-year planning plan of action and milestones (POA&M) is shown in Figure 4–6.

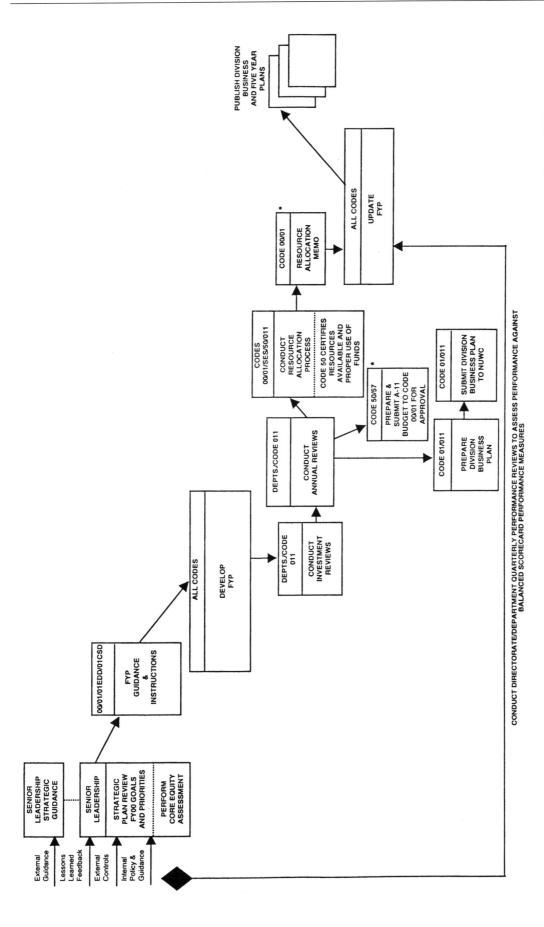

Figure 4–4. FY01–05 5-Year Planning Process. *Source:* Head, Strategy Development Staff (Code 011), Naval Undersea Warfare Center, Division Newport, Newport, Rhode Island.

• Prepare Planning Guidance and Instructions	Dec–Jan
• Release Guidance and Instructions	14 Feb
• Develop Five Year Plan (All Codes)	Feb–May
• Conduct Investment Reviews (Round 1)	1–10 Mar
• Division Investment Proposals Due to Support Investment Process	24 Mar
• Conduct Investment Reviews (Round 2)	1–10 Apr
• Finalize Approved Investment Projects & Request Additional Documentation	20 Apr
• Conduct the Annual Review (All Codes)	5 May
• Prepare Business Plan and A-11 Budget for Review & Approval (NUWCNPT and NUWC CM Review)	May–Jun
• Finalize Division Business Plan for Submission to NAVSEA	Jul
• Conduct Resource Allocation Process	1 Jul–20 Aug
• Issue Resource Allocation Memo	1 Sep
• Update to Five Year Plan Data	Sep–Nov
• Publish Five Year Plans	Dec
• Conduct Quarterly Performance Reviews	Oct–Jan–Mar–Jul

Figure 4–5. FY01–05 5-Year Planning Schedule. *Source:* Head, Strategy Development Staff (Code 011), Naval Undersea Warfare Center, Division Newport, Newport, Rhode Island.

	1st Qtr			2nd Qtr			3rd Qtr			4th Qtr		
	Oct	Nov	Dec	Jan	Feb	Mar	Apr	May	Jun	Jul	Aug	Sep
Final Division Business Plan/Document Core Equity Assessments/Sustainable Plan & Determine Investment Strategy		▲										
Prepare External Scan			▲——▲									
Release Guidance & Instructions					▲							
Directorate/Departments Develop Five Year Plans (All Codes)					△———————▲							
Investment Proposal Submissions Due to Code 011 (24 Mar)						△						
Finalize Approved Investment Projects & Request Additional Required Documentation (April)							△—△					
Directorate/Departments Submit Five Year Plans to Code 011								△				
Conduct the Division Annual Planning Review								△				
Prepare Division Buisness Plan and A-11 Budget for Review and Approval (May–Jun)*								△——△				
Conduct the Resource Allocation Process (Jun–Aug)									△————————△			
Finalize the Division Business Plan for Submission to NAVSEA (1 Jul)										△		
Issue the Resource Allocation Memo—Directorates/Departments To Update the Five Year Plans (8 Sep)*												△
FY01 Conduct Directorate/Department Performance Reviews—Quarterly	○		○			○			○			

*Includes NUWC TD & 00 Review.

Figure 4–6. FY01–05 5-Year Planning POA&M. *Source:* Head, Strategy Development Staff (Code 011), Naval Undersea Warfare Center, Division Newport, Newport, Rhode Island.

NEWSPAPER ARTICLE: FIVE-YEAR PLANNING EXPLAINED IN ONE EASY LESSON

The article that follows is reprinted from T. Edgar, "Five Year Planning Explained in One Easy Lesson," p. 5–6, *NUWSCOPE,* Vol. 30, No. 3., March 2000.

How NUWC Operates as a Business

In a recent conversation about key business processes that are used at the Newport Division, Juergen Keil, the Executive Director, noted, "the Division five-year planning process is one of the most important cornerstones of our Strategic Management Process." The use of the annual planning process to craft agreement between the Commander and Executive Director and the directorate and department heads on the future course of the Division and their departments "makes us fairly unique among government activities."

All departments and directorates use this defined and systematic process (see box), which has been in place since 1981, to develop program and management plans for a five-year-planning window. The plans are used to document a variety of data including strategies, resource requirements, and the skills needed to support the current Navy, the future Navy, and the Navy after next.

Annual five-year planning process review

External Scan—documents trends and events that could impact Newport Division business activity.

Guidance development and distribution—based on scan data, external guidance and internal survey results, and used to guide plan preparation.

Plan preparation and submission—departments develop program and management plans in accordance with guidance.

Annual plan review meeting—provides a Division-wide view of resource requirements and an opportunity to discuss issues and share information.

Plan analysis—plans and review-meeting data analyzed to support resource allocation decision process.

Resource allocation—allocates indirect and G&A, core equity, sustainment initiative and associated investment funds, and sets performance targets.

Plan execution—departments do what is planned

Performance measure—performance monitored at Quarterly Performance Reviews and with the Balanced Scorecard.

The five-year plans are aligned with other products of the Division's strategic management process. These include the mission, vision, operating principles, and goals contained in the Strategic Plan that define the long-term vision of where the Division is going and how it is going to get there. The five-year plans have a tactical focus that provides program initiative and resource utilization plans that enable near-term progress toward strategic goal and vision attainment. And the accumulation of funding and work year projections, in turn, provide valuable input in the preparation of the Division's annual A-11 budget submission and are used to formulate stabilized work year rate was explained in a September 1999 *NUWSCOPE* article; the budget process will be discussed in a future *NUWSCOPE* article.

The development this year of the Division's first business plan, prepared in response to NAVSEA direction, was able to capitalize on the sound work used in the development of the Division's FY00–04 five-year plans. This year's planning guidance, which will guide development of the FY01–05 plans, has been modified to bring our five-year plan development in close alignment with our business plan development. This alignment will minimize the preparation burden placed on Division employees.

Five-year Planning Process

The process begins in the first quarter of the fiscal year with an external scan that documents key trends and events that shape the USW environment and can influence Division business activity. The scan includes data on policy and regulatory trends, market analysis, long-term Navy needs and requirements, and a quick-look at socio-economic factors that could impact the Division over the planning period. Scan data are integrated with the results of the Customer Survey and Employee Opinion Survey and with a synthesis of Navy and DoD strategic plans and associated planning guidance. This information, together with guidance from the Technical Director of NUWC, is used to establish five-year planning guidance.

Distribution of the five-year planning guidance in the second quarter of the fiscal year initiates the planning process. The guidance tasks directorates and departments to develop a comprehensive plan addressing all elements of running their business area. This includes defining overall technical/functional program direction, goals, business initiatives, resource requirements, training plans, strategic skill requirements, environmental plans, investment needs, and metrics with quantifiable targets. For the FY01–05 plan cycle, departments will also address core equity sustainment, business base trends, workforce effectiveness initiatives, and customer loyalty initiatives. These additions strengthen the alignment of the five-year plans with the new business planning process. The guidance requires consideration of and planning for all aspects of near- and long-term direction and needs. Plan development involves discussion with other Division departments, customers, suppliers, and stakeholders in the formulation of realistic and challenging goals and robust plans for execution in the planning window.

How the Plans Are Used

Following their completion by the directorates and departments, the plans are reviewed during the Annual Plan Review meeting, which is usually conducted in May. It is led by the Commander and Executive Director and involves senior managers from all directorates and departments. The meeting provides a Division-wide view of resource requirements identified in the plans. The review meeting, which provides a forum in which important issues are identified and discussed, best practices are shared, and the management team is informed of key program challenges and opportunities, starts the process of building a Division-level picture of the future.

Resource allocation is the next step in the process. It is based on an analysis of the information developed during the annual plan review meeting, knowledge about externally imposed resource constraints and mandates, and negotiations between Division and directorate and department leaders. Resources allocated through this process include: overhead and service cost center budgets (indirect and G&A), Division training budget and plan, staffing levels (including hiring), core equity sustainment initiatives and associated investment funds, and facility maintenance projects. In addition, operating targets for direct work year performance and productivity ratio are established. The Commander and Executive Director normally release the resource allocation memorandum in August; it documents resource allocation decisions and establishes resource utilization policies for the next fiscal year.

Performance Measurement

The Division took the lead among Navy activities in linking performance measurement with the planning process in 1994 when it developed an enterprise-level system of performance measures. The measures selected—Customer, Employee/Learning and Growth, Financial, Internal Business, and Stakeholder—have become the Division's Balanced Scorecard (BSC). They are used as indicators of the overall organizational health and to assess progress toward achieving the strategic goals. The BSC approach to performance measurement is an integral part of the strategic management process and since the 1997 planning cycle each directorate and department has arrayed its key measures into the five perspectives of the BSC. Quarterly review of Division, directorate, and department BSC metrics are conducted and provide an opportunity to assess, and if necessary redirect, action needed to keep the Division moving toward goal attainment.

On a quarterly basis, performance against the plan and against operating targets is assessed during the Quarterly Performance Review (QPR) conducted by the Commander and Executive Director with directorate and department heads. QPRs also address program highlights, the BSC metrics, customer survey data, safety and environmental initiatives, and core equity sustainment initiatives.

Why Do We Do All of This . . .?

When asked, "Why do we do all of this planning? After all, plans and reality tend to diverge, especially in the out years," Keil responded: "The deliberative process that occurs during plan development and review provides value to our overall management process. We continue to use this systematic planning process because it enables a strategic conversation between Division leaders that prepares us to make smart business decisions based on consideration of a broad range of options that encompass customer, NAVSEA, and Navy concerns. By assessing future contingencies, articulating alternatives, and addressing resource requirements, the Division is better positioned to face organizational challenges and respond to them with coherent policies and plans." He concluded by saying that "documenting the plan development process and sharing it with the workforce helps to communicate business priorities and realities. The Five-Year Plans, together with the Division Strategic Plan and Business Plan, help employees understand where the Division is headed and how they can help the Division realize its goals."

So, if you have never read a Five-Year Plan, talk to your branch, division, or department head. Copies of previous years' plans are available in the Division's Technical Library. Business plan information was provided in articles in the January and February issues of *NUWSCOPE*. Your branch head soon will have a copy of the Business Plan that you can examine.

If you have questions or ideas about the annual five-year planning process, please contact Traci Edgar of the Corporate Strategy Development Staff.

CHAPTER 5

The Balanced Scorecard at the Veterans Benefits Administration

The Veterans Benefits Administration (VBA) is a major organization within the Department of Veterans Affairs. It also is responsible for one of the best implementations of the BSC in the federal government.

VBA has been developing its BSC concept for the past several fiscal years. In May 1998, VBA grouped all regional offices into nine geographically based service delivery networks (SDNs), which were established to provide mutual support and to share resources. The performance of the SDNs was recorded and assessed through the VBA's BSC, which standardized five performance categories across all of VBA's business lines. The categories are: (1) accuracy, (2) customer satisfaction, (3) employee development, (4) processing timeliness, and (5) cost. Accuracy is given the most weight among the five categories.

The material that follows reflects some of the complexity of implementing GPRA. It is a circular disseminating a revised process within VBA for the compensation and pension claims processing accuracy review processes and for compiling measurement data required by GPRA. This circular has been adapted for use here; more information is included in Appendix B to this book.

VBA used informal best practices learned among the various offices processing and issuing certificates to meet the timeliness requirements in the BSC.

SYSTEMATIC TECHNICAL ACCURACY REVIEW PROGRAM FOR COMPENSATION AND PENSION CLAIMS PROCESSING

The following material is adapted from the Veterans Benefits Administration, Department of Veterans Affairs, *Systematic Technical Accuracy Review Program for Compensation and Pension Claims Processing*, November 24, 1998, Circular 21-98-3.

Purpose

Compensation and pension claims processing accuracy review processes have been revised to standardize and improve the review process and to provide measurement data required by the Government Performance and Review Act (GPRA). This revised process, called Systematic Technical Accuracy Review (STAR), provides for reviews in three key processing areas (rating, authorization, and fiduciary work). The STAR program will be required for both national and local reviews to ensure consistent methodology for accuracy assessments at the national, service delivery network, and regional office level. This circular provides basic instructions for conducting, recording, and assessing STAR results.

Background

The STAR program reflects the recommendations of a special Quality Work Group formed to propose a revised accuracy review system, which would improve quality assurance methodology and support development of comprehensive GPRA measures. The Work Group reviewed current and prior C&P quality programs, quality assurance programs of peer organizations, and the recommendations provided in various reports including the Adjudication Claims Commission, National Association of Public Administrators (NAPA) report, as well as several General Accounting Office (GAO) reports and Inspector General (IG) studies.

The initial STAR plan was modified to reflect the performance measurement and organization changes outlined in VBA's *Roadmap to Excellence*, dated May 29, 1998. The *Roadmap to Excellence* plan grouped all regional offices into nine geographically based Service Delivery Networks (SDNs). The Service Delivery Networks were established to provide mutual support and share resources. The SDN plan envisions cooperative team-based collaborative leadership and shared collective accountability for overall SDN performance. The performance of the Service Delivery Networks will be recorded and assessed through VBA's Balanced Scorecard. This scorecard standardizes five performance categories across all of VBA's business lines. The categories are accuracy, customer satisfaction, employee development, processing timeliness, and unit cost.

Because all members of an SDN share responsibility and accountability for all of the work assigned to the Network, the Balanced Scorecard for each SDN and the national Balanced Scorecard will be the only formal and official measures of organizational performance by the Compensation and Pension Service. Measurement of accuracy (as with the other balanced scorecard components) will be focused at the Network level of performance. Assessment of accuracy at the SDN level will require statistically valid sampling and assessment of accuracy for each of the nine SDNs for each review area. Each SDN sample will be a stratified sample reflecting each regional office's relative share of its respective SDN's total completed workload for the prior fiscal year. The accuracy rate for the nation will be a compilation of the C&P Service review results for the nine SDNs weighted to reflect relative share of national workload.

STAR Program Overview

The STAR program includes three separate, but complementary program area reviews. Together, these reviews will assess all critical elements of claims adjudication. (Telephone and personal communication with claimants will be addressed in the balanced scorecard on the basis of customer satisfaction studies.) The three reviews of the STAR program include: core rating-related end products, core authorization end products, and fiduciary cases. Reviews to establish national and SDN level accuracy rates will be conducted by C&P Service. Reviews to assess regional office claims processing accuracy will be conducted locally.

Core Rating End Product Review

All elements covered by an end product subject to review will be considered in the review. If, during a review of a core rating end product case, a problem is identified with required authorization actions such as income or dependency issues, the error will be documented and the case will be considered "in error." The core rating–related end product review will include the following end products:

EP 010   Original Disability Compensation, 8 or more issues
EP 110   Original Disability Compensation, 1 to 7 issues
EP 180   Original Disability Pension
EP 140   Original DIC (Dependency & Indemnity Compensation)
EP 020   Reopened Disability Compensation
EP 120   Reopened Disability Pension
EP 070   Appeal Processing (Supplemental SOC & Certification)
EP 172   Appeal Statement of the Case (SOC)
EP 174   Hearing by Hearing Officer
EP 095   Vocational Rehabilitation Determination with Rating

Core Authorization End Product Review

The core authorization end product review will concentrate on authorization end products requiring significant development, review, and administrative decision or award action. Infrequently, some rating actions may be required for some of these end products. Any included rating action is also subject to review. The list of authorization end product areas subject to review includes:

EP 130   Dependency Adjustment or Decision
EP 135   Hospital Adjustment
EP 150   Income Related Adjustment or Decision
EP 155   EVR Related Adjustment or Decision
EP 160   Burial Related Decision
EP 165   Decision Involving Accrued Benefits
EP 190   Original Death Pension
EP 290   Misc. Eligibility Determinations
EP 600   Due Process

Review of Fiduciary Cases

A sample of Principal Guardianship Files (PGF) will be reviewed to monitor the accuracy of fiduciary work.

STAR Procedures

The STAR process requires a comprehensive review and analysis of all elements of processing associated with a specific claim. The STAR check sheets were designed to facilitate consistent structured reviews of claims. Only outcome related deficiencies should be recorded as errors. Such deficiencies include improper application of the not well-grounded rule, failure to address all issues, improper development, improper or inaccurate final decision on the claim, lack of proper notification, and failure to apply due process requirements. An error is only recorded if it was not corrected prior to finalization of the end product action. If a claim was not properly developed at the outset, but prior to award action and notification of the claimant, that deficiency was identified and corrected, a reportable error does not exist for STAR purposes. Procedural deficiencies unrelated to outcome will not be recorded as errors, but may be documented as a comment or remark. If a problem is identified with an issue not included in the claim (end product) under review, that problem should be documented as a remark or comment, but should not be recorded as an error. While comments or remarks will have no impact on the statistical assessment of accuracy, they will provide information for local management and in some cases assist a claimant.

For each folder reviewed, the case will be considered either correct or in error: i.e., it is either all right or it is wrong. An answer of "No" to any of the questions on the checklist relating to the processing of the claim (end product) action under review will result in the case being classified as "in error." (The last section of each checklist contains an area for administrative questions that are not related to the accuracy of claims processing; an answer of "No" for one of these questions will not indicate error in the case.)

If during review of a case no documented basis for the end product action subject to review is found, or the end product recorded was incorrect, the block for correct end product should be checked "No" on the review sheet and a formal review should not be conducted. (The third digit modifier will not be considered for purposes of establishing whether or not an end product subject to review is considered correct.) The facts concerning the end product discrepancy should be recorded as a comment or remark. Any other apparent discrepancies should also be recorded as a remark. An invalid end product will not be considered an error for STAR accuracy rate purposes, but the case will be excluded from the review sample. A substitute case listing will be generated by C&P Service for review.

Reviewers must be thorough in their review of each claim. It is not sufficient to simply review a decision and the letter of notification. All of the evidence associated with a claim must be reviewed to ensure that all issues (inferred as well as claimed) have been properly adjudicated. The general guideline for answering "No" to any question is the criteri[on] of irrefutable error. Judgment or difference of opinion reflecting a possible better practice or solution should be recorded as a comment or remark rather than an error. This does not mean that a decision based on an evaluation or weighing of evidence is exempt from a finding of error. Sound judgment is required and exercise of judgment must meet a "reasonable range" test. Resolution of reasonable doubt (evidence in equipoise—38 CFR 3.102) in a claimant's favor is mandated by regulation. Failure to properly apply 38 CFR 3.102 represents irrefutable error.

Sufficient narrative must be provided to clearly identify and explain the error called. In most cases the explanation for the error(s) found should be sufficient to allow a reader to understand the problem area(s) without reviewing the claims folder. While this is not possible for all cases, it is for most. If the correct action was something more than the obvious converse of the erroneous action, then a statement indicating what the correct action would have been is required. Appropriate citation supporting an error call must be provided. When possible, the reference should cite the appropriate statute or regulation, but it may also cite a Court of Veterans Appeals (COVA) precedent decision, General Counsel precedent decision, manual provision, circular, or fast letter. Do not cite material from informal communications, local instructional letters, training guides, etc.

Cascade Effect

Based on the logical progression of the review sheets, when an error is identified, generally all subsequent processing related to that issue will also be in error. For example, if an issue was not addressed, it is likely that the issue was not developed; it is most likely that the issue was not rated; and it is also most likely that notification for this issue was not sent. As a second example, if a claim was properly developed but not properly rated, then inherently, the notification would be incorrect. This pattern of derived error is referred to as a *cascade* effect. Recording additional errors inherent in the initial deficiency would distort identification of the basic or critical errors of the case, while adding little or no insight into root causes of the error itself. STAR reviews are outcome oriented and not process oriented. Once an error is found and recorded concerning a specific issue associated with a claim (i.e., a "No" answer for one of the processing questions), no additional errors related to that issue should be recorded. The review of the case must continue for any other issues subject to review and the first error found in processing each additional issue contained within the claim should be recorded. The additional errors found and documented will not change the outcome for the particular case—since any one critical error (a "No" answer) makes the whole case wrong. Documentation of additional critical errors, however, will provide valuable information about the nature of primary errors and a better definition of the extent of accuracy concerns for station or Service Delivery Network review (i.e., of the cases in error, how many total critical errors were identified and in what categories?). For cases involving only a single issue, "Not applicable" would be the appropriate answer for all the questions that follow the initial "No" answer.

National Reviews

C&P Service will perform national reviews to measure SDN and national accuracy. A specific staff within C&P Service has been developed and assigned this task. C&P Service will directly request cases subject to review from the regional office of jurisdiction. The regional offices will be responsible for promptly mailing the requested claims folders to C&P Service. The folders will be returned with individual case review results included upon completion of the review. The only acceptable reasons for not transferring a case for review include: folder transferred to BVA for appellate review; folder controlled for possible COVA review or transferred to the General Counsel for COVA review; or folder lost (circularized). If a folder has been transferred to another regional office, C&P Service should be notified of the transfer so that the folder can be requested from the regional office of current jurisdiction.

Annually, C&P Service will review 354 core rating-related cases, 325 authorization-related cases, and 140 fiduciary cases for each SDN. The sample size for rating and authorization cases are based on required 95 percent confidence factor and ± 5 percent margin of error for SDN accuracy rates. A critical factor in determining required sample size is the anticipated variation in the sample. Results of the two baseline reviews were used for this purpose. Required sample size increases with increased variation in the sample reviewed. Accordingly, a larger sample of rating cases is required based on baseline accuracy of 64 percent compared to the 70 percent baseline accuracy of authorization actions. Fiduciary reviews will be based initially on a judgment sample reflecting the relatively small share of overall workload that this category of work represents.

Reviews will be conducted on a quarterly basis to provide each SDN a sense of its accuracy status and, as appropriate, an indication when additional intervention may be required to meet accuracy goals. To distribute the workload and to minimize the frequency of stations transferring cases for review, three SDNs will be reviewed each month. Approximately 205 cases will be reviewed for each SDN for a total C&P Service monthly review workload of 615 cases.

Local Reviews

While the adoption of a unified and centralized accuracy program based on STAR assessments of SDN processing meets national and delivery network measurement and performance assessment requirements, it does not meet all process management requirements. Specifically, it does not provide accuracy information to a degree sufficient to independently assess the performance of each regional office and provide regional office specific information to regional office managers. A local review is necessary for this purpose. Local management must implement an active and comprehensive accuracy review program for self-assessment that will provide essential management information concerning training requirements and operational areas requiring additional management intervention. Each regional office is required to implement a local accuracy review consistent with the national review, utilizing the STAR process and procedures. SDN leadership must ensure that local reviews are done in a timely and accurate manner.

Local reviews must follow the . . . STAR checklists . . . for rating core end product work, . . . for authorization core end product work, and . . . for fiduciary cases. [See Appendix B.] These checklists were developed with the assistance and input of a panel of experienced subject matter experts, including a number of current field managers. These checklists represent a detailed and comprehensive analysis of claims processing performance in all key areas, viewed from a claims service perspective rather than a merely procedural perspective. Each station must conduct separate reviews of rating related end products, authorization end products, and fiduciary cases.

For rating and authorization, each station will be provided review lists based upon sample size required for statistically valid assessments (95% confidence level and ± 5% margin of error). For fiduciary, a judgment sample will be used. As with the SDN and national level review, the number of cases required to be reviewed each year may decrease with an improvement in the accuracy rate in subsequent years. Samples will be drawn by C&P Service from listings of the prior month's completed cases stored in the Austin database of completed cases. If local management desires an enhanced review to target particular areas of program issues or processing concern, additional cases may be reviewed based on locally generated samples. However, results of supplemental reviews must be maintained separately (and should not be recorded in the STAR database), since only reviews based on C&P generated lists will represent a valid random sample on which to base the local assessment of regional office accuracy.

Each month, C&P Service will send each regional office a list of cases to review. Those cases must be reviewed within 30 days except in exceptional circumstances. Each review list will represent 0th of a station's annual required reviews. All of the cases on the review list must be reviewed except for: cases transferred to BVA; transferred to the General Counsel for COVA review; invalid end products; or lost folders. A temporary transfer-in must be requested for folders on the review list that have been permanently transferred to another regional office. Reviews for cases temporarily unavailable because of transfer to a medical center for examination purposes should be completed upon return of the claim folder. At the end of each 30-day review period, a status report must be submitted electronically to the Office of Field Operations (VAVBAWAS/CO/OFO) indicating the status of the review. The status report should specifically identify cases excused from the review and separately list cases for which reviews will be delayed pending return of a folder. (This activity will be mostly automated when the STAR database is activated.) For cases excused from the review, substitute case listings will be provided by C&P Service.

Recording and Analysis of Review Results

The results of both local and national reviews will be maintained in a consolidated database. Useful reports will be available at a variety of levels, including national, SDN, and regional office. The results of the local reviews must be analyzed by regional office and SDN management to ensure that performance expectations are met, or, if not, that appropriate management and training steps are developed/implemented to ensure improvement. The reports generated from the local reviews will be indicators for the program managers, but *the official measure of accuracy for the SDN and the nation will be the results of the C&P Service reviews.* The SDNs, Office of Field Operations, and C&P Service will conduct regular meetings to discuss review results and to plan any necessary steps for improvement. If specific stations are identified as requiring assistance, Network management will work with C&P Service and Field Operations to develop improvement plans and to conduct supplemental reviews to assess results.

Until the database is available (and thoroughly tested), the accuracy findings of the stations' local reviews must be reported monthly to the Office of Field Operations (VAVBAWAS/ CO/OFO) with a copy to C&P Service, (VAVBAWAS/CO/214B). The database will be an intranet application accessible by all regional offices, Office of Field Operations, and C&P Service. A detailed user's guide will be provided upon completion and testing of the database.

Local Review Process Assessment

Various stakeholders have expressed considerable interest and support for the establishment of procedures to review and ensure the consistency and accuracy of local reviews. To provide a basis for assessing the local review process, C&P Service agreed to select for the national review, cases that had previously been subject to regional office review. The results of the two reviews will be compared to establish the adequacy of local reviews. The C&P review will not constitute a validation of the local accuracy rate, but rather an adequacy check of the review process. The number of cases reviewed for each regional office will be the number of cases required for national review based on the stratified sample for each SDN. An annual minimum of 25 cases each for rating and authorization will be reviewed for each regional office. (A formula will be applied when computing the SDN accuracy rate to weight the results of small station reviews proportionately to their share of SDN completed workload.) This procedure will begin with reviews conducted by C&P Service in January 1999. The first 2 month's reviews will be of an independent sample of cases to avoid delaying C&P reviews until completion of initial regional office reviews. All C&P reviews will be included in establishing SDN and national accuracy rates, but only the last 10 months of C&P reviews will be used to evaluate local review processes.

Office of Field Operations, SDN representatives, and C&P Service will monitor the results of the comparative reviews for the first half of FY 1999, before defining an acceptable range of performance. Individual case reviews will be considered consistent if both reviews either find no errors, or both find an error. If a regional office's review ultimately does not meet the acceptable range, an independent review of a statistically valid sample of cases may be conducted by the SDN with the assistance of the Office of Field Operations and C&P Service. The results of that review would be considered the regional office's official accuracy rate.

Dispute Resolution

It is anticipated that occasionally regional offices may receive a review result with which they disagree or believe the explanation offered is unclear or inadequate. For instances of simple clarification, telephone inquiries to the Chief of the C&P Review Staff (Bill Bauer (202) 273-7274) are always welcome. However, any basic disagreement over the correctness of a call must be formally addressed. If a regional office believes an erroneous call has been made, the case may be returned for a formal determination by the Director of Compensation and Pension Service. To request reconsideration, a memorandum to the Director of Compensation and Pension Service must be prepared stating the basis for the request for reconsideration. The memorandum should include pertinent supporting statute, regulation, COVA, GC Opinion, or manual citations. The claim folder should be submitted with the memorandum for review. The regional office will be provided a formal decision. Results of reconsideration requests will be maintained and monitored to ensure the effectiveness and integrity of the review process.

Finally, regional offices should notify the Director, C&P Service, if they have concerns about the tone and/or content of review narratives even if the regional office otherwise agrees with the merits of the exception.

Robert J. Epley
Director, Compensation and Pension Service

CHAPTER 6

Balanced Measures at the Internal Revenue Service

The Internal Revenue Service (IRS) has one of the broadest implementations of the Balanced Scorecard in the federal government. As the commissioner of the IRS embarked on the massive management and leadership task of turning the IRS around, he explained how he was going to modernize the IRS and significantly improve tax service to the American public.

Appearing before the Senate Finance Committee on January 28, 1998, he discussed the new mission of the agency. He stated that the modernized IRS would be guided by five principles. One of these five principles was to use Balanced Measures of performance. Prior to these changes, the system focused on IRS internal operations and failed to account for the taxpayers' viewpoint and satisfaction. The new Balanced Measures will take into account: (1) overall compliance by major taxpayer segment, (2) customer satisfaction, (3) employee satisfaction, and (4) continuous improvement.

The next several pages contain an excerpt from the commissioner's statement before the Senate Finance Committee and the goals of the IRS for the year 2000. A very detailed segment on the IRS Balanced Measurement System follows; it is adapted from the Internal Revenue Manual (IRM) 105.4. This application is somewhat unique in the federal government for several reasons. First, the entire agency of more than 100,000 personnel is subject to it. Second, Balanced Measures is one of the five levers of change for modernizing the IRS. Third, the measurement system focuses on what is important to achieve the strategic goals of the IRS. Therefore, the alignment of the measurement system with the mission of the IRS is impressive in the upper echelons of the federal government. Fourth, dollar measures of performance are not part of the measurement system. Finally, there is no ranking of offices.

The chapter concludes with a new document, *Organizational Performance Management and the IRS Balanced Measurement System,* released in June 2000. It presents an update on the IRS Balanced Measurement System.

The IRS Balanced Measurement System elements are customer satisfaction, employee satisfaction, and business results. Business results consist of quality, quantity, and outreach. The IRS material is rich in detail on what the system is and what the system is not. The material provides much insight into why the system is used and what the IRS commissioner is trying to achieve in modernizing the IRS.

COMMISSIONER'S TESTIMONY

The following material is adapted from *Statement of Charles O. Rossotti, Commissioner of Internal Revenue, Before the Senate Finance Committee, January 28, 1998,* www.irs.gov.

A Modernized IRS

Commissioner of Internal Revenue Charles O. Rossotti has developed a concept of a modernized American tax agency that will deliver significantly improved service to American taxpayers. The modern Internal Revenue Service will focus on the taxpayer's understanding and solving problems from the taxpayer's point of view. The new mission for the agency should be to help people comply with the law and ensure fairness of compliance.

The modernized IRS will be guided by five principles: understand and solve problems from the taxpayer's point of view, expect managers to be accountable, use balanced measures of performance, foster open, honest communications, and insist on total integrity.

The Goals of a Modernized IRS Will Reflect the New Focus on Taxpayers as Customers

Service to each taxpayer. The IRS will continue to make filing easier and provide first quality service to every taxpayer needing help. Taxpayers who may owe additional taxes or cannot pay what they owe will receive prompt, professional, helpful treatment.

Service to all taxpayers. The IRS will serve the American taxpaying public by increasing overall compliance and by increasing the fairness of compliance programs.

Productivity through a quality work environment. The IRS will increase employee job satisfaction and hold agency employment stable while the economy grows and service improves.

Achieving a Modernized IRS Will Require Significant Changes in Five Separate Areas

Revamped business practices. Business practices will be geared toward understanding, solving, and preventing taxpayer problems. Much greater emphasis will be placed on customer education and service. Compliance efforts will be forward looking to prevent most common taxpayer problems and will be geared toward early intervention to keep taxpayers compliant. Compliance tools will be reserved for only those who refuse to comply and will be used more sparingly.

Four operating units. Much of the current national office and regional office structures will be realigned to form management teams, each with end-to-end responsibility for serving a group of taxpayers with like needs. The four groups are: individual taxpayers with wage and investment income, small business and self-employed taxpayers, large business taxpayers, and employee plans/exempt organizations and state and local governments. Each organizational unit will have a tailored set of services to meet the needs of the taxpayers served by that unit. This organizational model, based on similar models in private industry, provides for fewer managerial layers and clear lines of responsibility. Currently, IRS managers are often responsible for administering the entire Internal Revenue Code across the full spectrum of taxpaying customers. Managers in the new business units will be able to focus on the specific needs of the taxpayers they serve.

Balanced measures of performance. Current IRS performance measures are oriented toward IRS internal operations and fail to account for the taxpayers' viewpoint and satisfaction. The new measures will be externally validated and will entail a balanced scorecard tied to the agency's goals. The new measures will take into account: overall compliance by major taxpayer segment, customer satisfaction, employee satisfaction, and continuous improvement.

Management roles with clear responsibility. By organizing around taxpayers with similar needs and issues, the management team for each of the four operating business units will be able to learn a great deal about the particular needs and problems affecting that group and be responsible for resolving those problems. The number of management layers in these new units will be fewer than the current levels of management, facilitating the implementation of new ideas, solutions, and better communications.

New technology. To support this business approach, the IRS is committed to move forward on upgrading and improving its technology through central, professional management, the establishment of common standards, and partnerships between the business units, the information technology professionals, and outside contractors.

The IRS plans to initiate a study to validate the concept for modernization and to plan for the implementation of the final plan. The study will involve extensive consultation with those involved with tax administration in this country both inside and outside the Internal Revenue Service. The IRS hopes to have this study phase done by this summer.

Improve Customer Satisfaction and Customer Service

The Internal Revenue Service (IRS) Customer Service Task Force found that our customers want fair, respectful, and courteous treatment; minimum contact with the IRS; easier, simpler forms and notices; easy access to help; and quick resolution of problems. In order to determine how we are doing, we developed customer satisfaction surveys for the major IRS business lines.

Goals
- Evaluate the results of the Customer Satisfaction Surveys for Fiscal Year (FY) 1999 and utilize these results to create measures of customer satisfaction for IRS and its major business lines as part of the balanced scorecard of performance.
- Minimize contacts with the IRS by rewriting by the end of FY 1999 the most frequently used taxpayer notices under the direction of a "notice gatekeeper."

Currently, the IRS processes over 215 million individual and business tax returns, with most of these transactions taking place on paper. The steady progress of the award-winning TeleFile program and other Electronic Tax Administration (ETA) initiatives gives a hint of the potential of electronic filing: less paper, no mail, an accuracy rate of 99 percent, faster refunds, and satisfied customers.

Goals
- Work toward making electronic filing truly paperless by piloting signature alternatives in FY 1999 and providing electronic payment options to taxpayers starting with Automated Clearing House (ACH) debit payments for balance due returns in FY 1999.
- Support and motivate the more than 85,000 Electronic Returns Originators (EROs) who provide electronic filing products and services to taxpayers and continue IRS' E-FILE campaign to better inform taxpayers and practitioners about the benefits of electronic filing. For FY 1999, increase the number of electronically filed individual returns filed through EROs to 21 million. Increase the number of individuals filing returns by phone (TeleFile) to over 6.6 million, which represents almost 27 percent of the 24.6 million taxpayers that are eligible to use this method of filing.
- If a complete and accurate tax return is filed and a taxpayer is due a refund, the IRS will issue a refund within 21 days if it was electronically filed and within 40 days if filed as a paper return.

Provide Better Telephone Service

The IRS runs one of the nation's most heavily used 800-number operations. In FY 1997, nearly 117 million callers reached the IRS by phone, up from 110.8 million in 1996 and 100.9 million in 1995.

Goals
- To make it easier for taxpayers to reach us, expand telephone service to 24 hours a day, 7 days a week by January 1, 1999. The IRS' goal is to provide this service with an access rate that will range from 85 percent to 90 percent for taxpayers calling the IRS and a tax law accuracy rate of 96 percent. We are currently working to improve our measurements for level of access and tax law accuracy. These measures will be revised and inserted here in the future.

Help Small Businesses

Small businesses are the fastest growing part of the national economy, and currently represent the overwhelming percent of all business tax returns. They are also the nation's largest private employer, accounting for 53 percent of private sector jobs and are the backbone of the wage reporting and withholding system. Everyone stands to gain by making it easier for them to fulfill their tax obligations.

Goals
- By the end of FY 1998, expand TeleFile to let many small businesses use their telephones to file quarterly federal tax returns and report employment taxes. In FY 1999, the IRS expects 1.2 million of an estimated 16 million eligible quarterly forms (Form 941) will be filed through TeleFile.
- To provide specialized products and services, especially in the area of electronic services for small businesses.

THE IRS BALANCED MEASUREMENT SYSTEM

The material that follows is adapted from Internal Revenue Service, "Chapter 2—The IRS Balanced Measurement System: A New Approach to Measuring Organizational Performance," in *Managing Statistics in a Balanced Measurement System,* Washington, D.C., Internal Revenue Service, September 15, 1999, Internal Revenue Manual 105.4.

[105.4] 2.1 (09-15-1999)

Overview

1) This chapter provides an overview of the IRS Balanced Measurement System and outlines how balanced measures, one of the five levers of change for modernizing the IRS, will be used to support a new approach to measuring organizational performance. This new measurement system focuses on what is important to achieve our strategic goals. The aim is to improve those processes that will make a difference. Dollar measures of

performance are not part of Balanced Measures and there will be no ranking of offices. The new organizational review process will be more forward-looking and will focus on actions taken to improve performance, not just the numeric measures results, i.e., the "numbers."

[105.4] 2.2 (09-15-1999)

What Is the IRS Balanced Measurement System?

1) The IRS Balanced Measurement System provides a means to:
   - Communicate organizational priorities, and better define what we need to focus upon as an organization.
   - Guide and motivate performance, and establish a linkage between performance goals and the organizational objectives.
   - Obtain feedback that will help us ascertain how well we are doing in meeting customer and stakeholder expectations and identify areas for improvement.

2) The elements of the Balanced Measurement System are Customer Satisfaction, Employee Satisfaction, and Business Results, with business results being comprised of measures of Quality and Quantity and Outreach. Each element represents an important aspect of the organization's goals and each is of equal importance in carrying out the Service's programs and functions. As such, any activity involving balanced measures, such as setting goals, assessing progress and evaluating results, must consider and address all elements of the Balanced Measurement System. Because some of these elements do not change as rapidly as others or require more time for data collection, the frequency of measures data availability may vary across the three elements. **However, such differences in the frequency of data availability do not reflect differences in priority.**

[105.4] 2.3 (09-15-1999)

Goals of the Balanced Measures Elements

1) The goals of the Balanced Measure elements are:
   - The goal of the Customer Satisfaction element is to provide accurate and professional services to internal and external customers in a courteous, timely manner.
   - The goal of the Employee Satisfaction element is to create an enabling work environment for employees by providing quality leadership, adequate training, and effective support services.
   - The goal of the Business Results element is to generate a productive quantity of work in a quality manner and to provide meaningful outreach to all customers.

2) Balanced Measures will be the measures used by the IRS to assess organizational performance at both the strategic level and the operational level. At the strategic level, such measures will be used to assess our overall performance in delivering on the mission and three strategic goals. Strategic measures would apply to the organization as a whole and to each of the major operating divisions in the modernized IRS. At the operational management level, measures are used to assess the effectiveness of program and service delivery of particular aspects of the organization, such as Customer Service, Collection, or Examination in the current organizational structure.

| | Balanced Measures | | | |
| | Customer Satisfaction | Employee Satisfaction | Business Results | |
			Quality	Quantity
Purpose/Goal	To serve customers professionally	To provide an enabling work environment	To do quality work	To work productively and to engage in proactive outreach activities designed to provide or enhance "top quality service" to all customers

[105.4] 2.4 (09-15-1999)

The Shift to Balanced Measures

1) The Balanced Measurement System has been developed as part of the effort to modernize the IRS and to reflect the Service's priorities, as articulated in the mission statement. This new approach to measurement will help shift the focus of individuals and the organization away from achieving a specific target or number to achieving the overall mission and strategic goals of the IRS.

2) Under the Balanced Measurement System, the IRS will still have and use performance results ("numbers"), but it will use these results much differently than it has in the past. Experience has shown that successful organizations cannot be managed by numbers alone. The numbers are only an indicator of past performance and, when considered by themselves, do not provide a complete picture of what is happening throughout the organization. IRS experience with various programs dealing with numerical performance goals over the past 40 years has shown that placing emphasis on one type of numeric goal can have an adverse impact on other important Service goals, e.g., productivity, quality case work, fair treatment of taxpayers, or employee satisfaction. The challenge given to the IRS through the Restructuring and Reform Act of 1998 was to develop an improved method of measuring performance that protects taxpayer rights, fosters quality service and considers the impact on employees. The Balanced Measurement System represents the IRS' response to that challenge.

[105.4] 2.5 (09-15-1999)

Balanced Measures and the IRS Management Model

1) The Service's management model represents a clear approach to managing our business and is directly linked to our mission, goals, and the Balanced Measurement System. The model is comprised of four elements: Plan, Do, Review, and Revise.

Elements of the Management Model

Plan: The "Plan" element "sets the strategy" and communicates areas of emphasis and what we will achieve with available resources. The Plan establishes clear direction, priorities, and goals. Balanced Measures are included in the plan as indicators of where we want to go and will help answer the question, "How will I know if I've achieved that strategy?"

Do: The "Do" element is the "day-to-day management" of activities.

Review: The "Review" element assesses the activities performed during "Do" against the

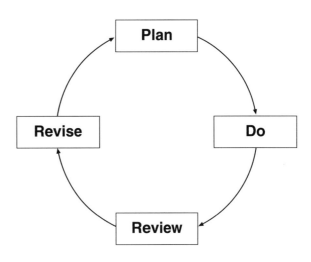

plan. Emphasis will be on actions taken to achieve objectives as each manager "looks behind the numbers." The review focuses on conducting detailed analysis to identify the root causes of changes in performance and to determine appropriate corrective actions.

Revise: In the "Revise" element, measures and actions are modified based upon the reviews.

2) We are not managing programs to achieve numbers; we are managing processes and people to achieve the IRS mission. Hence, using the Management Model, managers should collaborate with employees in developing plans, reviewing progress, and revising action plans.

[105.4] 2.6 (09-15-1999)

Using Balanced Measures

1) The new Balanced Measurement System will enable the Service to:
   - Measure how an organizational unit has performed relative to its past performance.
   - Identify areas that need action to help improve performance, taking all the measures—Customer Satisfaction, Employee Satisfaction, and Business Results—into consideration.
   - Align and support various review processes so that there is communication throughout the organization.
   - Begin a dialogue between managers and employees that is focused on discovering and positively impacting the factors that influence performance.
   - Provide input to managerial performance appraisals, not serve as a direct evaluative tool.
2) For an example of the Balanced Measures identified for use in Examination, Collection, and Customer Service, see Exhibit 105.4.2–3.

[105.4] 2.7 (09-15-1999)

Diagnostic Tools

1) The IRS collects a great deal of additional information about programs and services, some of which had been used as performance measures in the past. Under the Balanced

Measurement System, only the approved set of balanced measures—both strategic and operational—will be used to measure organizational performance. NO OTHER INFORMATION OR DATA WILL BE USED AS MEASURES OF ORGANIZATIONAL PERFORMANCE. Indicators that are not designated as "Balanced Measures," hereafter referred to as "diagnostic tools," will be used to help analyze the factors that affect changes in the balanced performance measures in order to "get behind the numbers." The use of diagnostic tools provides a mechanism to analyze factors that influence performance and encourages dialogue about specific actions that can be taken by managers to improve customer satisfaction, employee satisfaction, and business results. No goals or targets will be set for diagnostic tools nor will they be used in individual performance evaluations.

[105.4] 2.7.1 (09-15-1999)

Examples of Diagnostic Tools

2) . . . Diagnostic tools can include any type of data that is helpful in understanding what influences and impacts the balanced measures. In addition, it is permissible to use ROTERs as diagnostic tools. **In some cases, data used as a diagnostic tool for one organizational unit (i.e., cycle time) may be used as a balanced measure for a different organizational unit, and vice versa, as long as the measure conforms to the guidelines and restrictions set forth in Chapter 1.** A Reference Guide of Diagnostic Tools has been developed for Examination, Collection and Customer Service and this guidance is included in the respective functional chapters of IRM 105.4. However, the overall framework for the diagnostic tools translates to all functions and the guidance already provided for the Customer Satisfaction and Employee Satisfaction elements is relevant across most functions.

3) Diagnostic Tool Examples
   - ROTERs (Records of Tax Enforcement Results)
   - Results for individual questions on customer satisfaction surveys
   - Results for individual questions on employee satisfaction surveys
   - Cycle time
   - Employee experience/training/skill levels (i.e., hours of training per employee, workforce mix, average educational attainment of newly hired employees)
   - External factors (i.e., tax law, status of the economy)
   - Employee absenteeism, turnover rates
   - Physical resources
   - Work policies
   - Return closures per unit of effort
   - Inventory level
   - Survey rate
   - Examined return disposition mix
   - Workload mix
   - No change rate
   - Staffing resources (FTE appropriated, FTE realized, resource utilization)
   - Results for individual quality standards/elements
   - Wait time/transaction time
   - Cost information

[105.4] 2.7.2 (09-15-1999)

How Not To Use the Diagnostic Tools

1) Examples of how not to use the diagnostic tools
   - Do not use diagnostic tools as performance measures
   - Do not set goals or targets for diagnostic tools
   - Do not use as individual performance measures (e.g., in an individual performance evaluation)
   - Do not use diagnostic tools for evaluative comparisons with other units. Use them to understand underlying factors that cause changes in the Balanced Measures

[105.4] 2.3 (09-15-1999)

Setting Goals/Plan Development

1) The IRS' traditional use of performance measures and goals has changed significantly with the introduction of the Balanced Measurement System. Balanced performance measures and goals will no longer be used as stand-alone evaluative tools. Instead, these performance measures and results will serve as indicators of progress the IRS is making organizationally in achieving its strategic goals and mission. They will be used to assess and refine the actions taken to improve customer satisfaction, employee satisfaction, and business results.

2) The establishment of goals and the development of plans must consider and address all elements of the Balanced Measurement System—Customer Satisfaction, Employee Satisfaction, and Business Results.

3) *Individual managerial or employee evaluations will not be directly tied to balanced measures results. Non-managerial evaluations will be based upon critical elements or performance standards as appropriate and the review of work performed. Managerial evaluations will be based on the actions taken in accordance with an agreed upon plan and performance standards. For managers responsible for an organizational component, the quantitative measurements of the balanced measurement system are one of the factors that should inform a performance appraisal. They are not to be used as a stand-alone evaluative tool. (Note: *This guidance does not apply to the "Pipeline" area of Submission Processing where individual quality/quantity information is used consistent with existing work agreements.)

4) There are two types of goals an organization can use to communicate priorities and guide performance, *qualitative and quantitative. Qualitative goals are general in nature and suggest a desired direction but do not establish a numeric target, e.g., "Improve Customer Satisfaction." Quantitative goals, hereafter referred to as numeric goals, are specific and do establish a specific numeric target, e.g., "Improve Customer Satisfaction from 70 Percent to 80 Percent." As the IRS makes the migration to the Balanced Measurement System, the goals used by the organization will tend initially to be more *qualitative than quantitative. As data become available for the new measures and as the organization begins to understand and adapt to the balanced approach, goals will then become more quantitative. (Note: *The term "qualitative" is not the same as the Quality measure in Business Results. "Qualitative" *describes the type of goal, not the type of measure.* For example, a qualitative goal for the Business Results Quality measure might be "Improve the Accuracy of Tax Law Information Provided to Taxpayers." A quantitative/numeric goal for the Business Results Quality measure might be, "Improve the Tax Law Accuracy Rate from 85 Percent to 90 Percent.")

5) Quantitative and numeric goals will be set for the balanced measures at the Service wide level to satisfy requirements of the Government Performance and Results Act and other legislation. They will be used by the Service to report on Agency progress in delivering its tax administration responsibilities. Additional numeric goals will be set no lower than the District/Division level to be used primarily for planning purposes. They cannot and will not be used to directly determine the evaluations of either organizational units or individuals. Qualitative goals, however, can be established down to the group level for use in Action Plans established during the formal plan development process.

6) Performance measures results and diagnostic tools will be used to analyze and track program progress and improvements against both quantitative and qualitative goals. Managers and employees are expected to use this information for planning purposes and for making revisions to actions that have been identified in support of the various goals.

[105.4] 2.9 (09-15-1999)

Using the Numbers

1) The Balanced Measurement System is about changing the way the organization uses numbers; it is not about eliminating the use of numbers. Without numbers, it would be very difficult to effectively manage the Service or gauge progress in meeting our tax administration responsibilities. However, unlike most other organizations, the work performed by the IRS has the potential to substantially impact the lives of citizens as well as their trust in government. As government employees entrusted with ensuring the public good, it is the responsibility of each employee to make certain that taxpayer rights are upheld and protected. For these reasons, the IRS must exercise great care and caution in how it uses measures and "numbers." It cannot support a business and management approach focused only on the achievement of certain numbers and targets. Past behaviors and practices that may have contributed to such an approach have to change. The Balanced Measurement System has been designed to help employees, both managerial and non-managerial, actively engage in an approach to management and measurement at the IRS that is focused on identifying and taking appropriate actions to improve performance and on diagnosing the underlying factors that have influenced organizational outcomes. Following is an explanation of how the use of numbers will change under the Balanced Measurement System.

[105.4] 2.10 (09-15-1999)

Setting Goals

1) Goals for organizational performance measures will be set under the Balanced Measures framework in the areas of Customer Satisfaction, Employee Satisfaction, and Business Results. However, numeric goals will be set only to the levels for which statistically valid results are available for all components of the Balanced Measurement System—currently to the District (Center)/Division level. Numeric goals for each measure should be set in consideration of the other balanced measures and established based on a review of previous year results, the anticipated mix of resources available, and the linkage to organizational priorities and initiatives. At levels below the District (Center)/Division level, only qualitative goals, such as "Improve Case Quality," can be established for the balanced measures and would then include a set of specific actions.

[105.4] 2.11 (09-15-1999)

Communicating/Sharing Goals and Results

1) As data requirements are met for all elements of the Balanced Measurement System, Service wide numeric and qualitative goals will be included in organizational documents that are distributed broadly both within and outside the organization such as the budget submission, the annual performance plan, and the Operations plan. As such, Service wide qualitative goals can be shared and discussed at all levels of the organization with both managerial and non-managerial employees. Service wide numeric goals, however, should only be shared and discussed with managerial and non-managerial employees when there is a legitimate business purpose for sharing such data, such as the organizational planning process. **In any instance when numeric organizational goals are shared, caution must be exercised to ensure that any such discussion does not imply or suggest numeric goals for an individual or organization.**

2) District (Center)/Division qualitative goals can be shared at all levels of the organization. **District (Center)/Division numeric goals, however, should only be shared and discussed with managerial employees at the levels for which there is a legitimate business purpose for sharing such data,** i.e., at the branch level for planning purposes. Furthermore, District (Center) Directors and Division Chiefs must exercise great caution in how they share numeric goals in order to avoid the numbers focused pressures that were felt under previous measurement systems and to ensure that any such discussion does not imply or suggest numeric goals for that branch. Such sharing of goals should be done in a way that *does not* encourage the competitive environment that existed previously among some organizational units whose efforts were directed at achieving numeric targets without carefully considering the impact on all elements of the Balanced Measurement System—Customer Satisfaction, Employee Satisfaction, and Business Results.

3) Determining the appropriateness of sharing a goal depends on whether there is a good business reason for using such a statistic. Consider the following when making this decision:
   - What is the business reason for communicating the Goal?
   - What is the business risk of not providing the Goal?
   - What is the potential undesirable outcome that could come from the misuse of the Goal?
   - What is the risk that the intended recipient would reasonably believe that the communication suggested a quota or goal below the District (Center)/Division level or for an individual? Regarding this last element, consider:
     A) The degree of organizational knowledge and understanding of the intended recipient(s)
     B) The organizational climate at the time and place of the communication
     C) The context in which the communication is to be made
     D) Any guidance on how the Goal can or cannot be used
     E) The manner in which the communication is delivered
     F) The expectation of follow-up with respect to the Goal and the nature of the expected follow-up
     G) The probable internal perception of the communication of the Goal
     H) The probable public perception of the communication of the Goal

4) Under this approach, it would be allowable for a District (Center) Director or Division Chief to share numeric goals with Branch managers for use in the development of action plans as long as that discussion covered all components of the balanced measures and was done as part of the organizational planning process. For example, in any given

year, the organization's need to balance performance across all elements of the measures may require greater emphasis on some elements and lesser emphasis on other elements so as to maintain balance. This information is directly helpful in developing the supporting action plans and determining the types of actions necessary to achieve balance.

5) Once the action plans are completed, results should be looked at periodically because the numbers serve as indicators of the impact that actions are having on organizational performance. The discussions that must follow, however, need to focus on the specific actions, the extent to which it seems they are working and whether there is a need to revise or recommend additional actions. **It would never be appropriate for a District (Center) Director or Division Chief to use any discussion of numeric goals or results as an opportunity to apportion, establish, or suggest additional numeric goals at the branch or group levels.** And, once again, caution must be exercised in any such discussion to ensure that numeric goals for individuals are neither implied nor suggested.

6) *Sharing Data*—In sharing data/results for balance measures, the following restriction applies. Under the Balanced Measurement System, an organizational unit is allowed to see its own results (data) and the results of organizational units at levels above and below (if applicable). An organizational unit is not allowed to see results that are identifiable to other units at the same organizational level. This restriction is intended to help eliminate the competitive environment that existed in some areas among groups, branches, and districts to achieve the highest numeric results without considering the appropriateness of the actions being taken or the impact of those actions on each of the elements of the Balanced Measurement System. **Furthermore, the performance of any one unit at any level of the organization should not be used as a standard by which the performance of any other unit would be evaluated.** The appropriate purpose for sharing balanced measures results and diagnostic tool data among organizational units is in conducting analysis, identifying potential areas for improvement, and exploring best practices.

[105.4] 2.12 (09-15-1999)

Evaluating Performance of an Organizational Unit

1) In evaluating the performance of an organizational unit, the numeric results achieved with any of the balanced measures can be communicated orally and in writing in an organizational review only to the level for which numeric goals were established for all components of the Balanced Measurement System, i.e., currently the District (Center)/ Division level. Furthermore, at any time an organizational review is conducted, all components of the Balanced Measurement System must be considered and addressed. The inclusion of numeric results in an organizational review is only to provide a point of reference for a more detailed discussion of the impact of the actions that were taken to help achieve the IRS' mission and strategic goals as translated through the balanced measures. The reason for this restriction is to reduce the chance that the numeric results would be seen as the determining factor behind positive or negative organizational reviews, a situation that might cause the organization to regress to previous practices where organizational goals were inappropriately translated into individual goals.

2) Under this approach, it would be appropriate for an organizational review document for a Region or District (Center)/Division to display the numeric goals and results as long as they were provided in conjunction with a detailed discussion of the actions that

were taken to improve performance and, as appropriate, an explanation of the factors that may have influenced the final outcome. **It would not be appropriate for an organizational review to include specific measures results for organizational units below the District (Center)/Division level because no corresponding quantitative goals would be available from which the basis for such a numeric comparison could be made.** The discussions at those levels must be focused on action plans and related accomplishments, not numeric results.

[105.4] 2.13 (09-15-1999)

Evaluating the Performance of an Individual

1) In evaluating performance of an individual, the numeric results achieved with any of the balanced measures will never directly equate to the evaluation of any individual. Rather, a managerial evaluation must focus on the actions that were taken to improve performance in each area of the balanced measures. The numeric results are helpful only for making an initial assessment of the impact that those actions had on the balanced measures. The reason for this restriction is fundamental to the entire intent of the balanced measures approach and critical to changing behaviors. If individuals are held accountable solely for achieving specific numeric targets, the natural response is to focus attention on the numbers and not actions.

2) Using this guidance, it would be inappropriate for any written evaluation or performance discussion of an individual to reference a specific number, e.g., "John Smith, the Division Chief in District X, met the performance goals established in his performance plan. His office closed 500 more cases than the goal." An appropriate reference might be "John Smith, the Division Chief in District X, met the performance goals established in his performance plan. The agreed upon actions resulted in improvements in customer satisfaction, employee satisfaction, and business results." This overview would then be followed by a more detailed description of the specific actions that were taken toward achieving the goals.

[105.4] 2.14 (09-15-1999)

Day to Day Management

1) While numeric balanced measures goals will not be set below the District (Center)/Division level, numeric results for some of the balanced measures will be reported and statistically valid down to the branch level. The purpose for sharing numeric results at lower levels of the organization is to assist managers in the planning process, determine the impact actions are having on performance, and establish revised plans based on what is learned from the seven step process (see Section 2.15) to "get behind the numbers." Therefore, balanced measures results can be communicated throughout the organization when they are being used for an appropriate business purpose. However, in sharing results, the following restriction applies. Under the Balanced Measurement System, an organizational unit is allowed to see its own results and the results of organizational units at levels above and below (if applicable). An organizational unit is not allowed to see the results of other units at the same organizational level. This restriction is intended to help eliminate the competitive environment that existed in some areas among groups, branches, and districts to achieve the highest numeric results without

considering the appropriateness of the actions being taken or the impact of those actions on each of the elements of the Balanced Measurement System.

2) For example, a Division Chief completes a review of results for the balanced performance measures and observes that the Division is improving in the quality, customer satisfaction, and employee satisfaction areas but is experiencing declines in the quantity area. It would be appropriate for the Division Chief to meet with the Branch Chiefs and engage in a discussion about the performance of that Division and include references to the numeric results that have been achieved at the Division level. To make that discussion useful, the Division Chief could share trend information for the Division level results so that the Branch Chiefs can see the changes in performance for each balanced measure relative to the last data collection period, the previous year, etc. The focus of that discussion, however, must be on the actions taken and on "getting behind the numbers." The Division Chief might then say, "The action plans we established for our division are yielding positive results and are helping us meet our qualitative goals of improving customer satisfaction, employee satisfaction, and quality. However, we are experiencing a decline in quantity in comparison to the last quarter and in comparison to this time period last year even though we have the same mix of staffing and other resources. What do you think may be influencing this balanced measure element and how might we revise our plans to improve performance in this area?" **It would not be appropriate at any level, however, for a manager to distribute spreadsheets containing the balanced measures goals and monthly results to subordinate managers and then direct them to "improve performance."** Also, while the Division Chief would review the results of each branch for management purposes (e.g., to identify areas in which to focus attention, to identify best practices), the Division Chief should not share the numeric results of one branch with the others. If a best practice has been identified, it is allowable and encouraged for the Division Chief to share that practice with the other branches.

[105.4] 2.15 (09-15-1999)

Getting Behind the Numbers

1) Using balanced measures, "getting behind the numbers" is a seven step problem solving process as outlined below. Throughout this process, keep in mind that numbers are only a starting point and that, through analysis, implementation of a revised course of action is the objective.

[105.4] 2.15.1 (09-15-1999)

Receive Data

1) The first step is to obtain data. Data may be obtained from a variety of sources, examples of which are performance measures results (i.e., survey results, Quality Review Results, data on EMSS (Executive Management Support System)), data collected by the Taxpayer Advocate, and Diagnostic Indicators. In other instances, data may have to be locally developed.

[105.4] 2.15.2 (09-15-1999)

Define the Problem

1) In some cases, the problem may be obvious. In other cases, you will need to analyze the data to identify the problem.
2) If you suspect a problem, then ask the question, "What is the real problem?"
3) State the problem in objective terms. An accurately worded problem statement is important for the other steps in the process.
4) A good example is: "Taxpayers do not have a sufficient understanding of IRS procedures." Not: "IRS employees are not explaining our procedures sufficiently to taxpayers."

[105.4] 2.15.3 (09-15-1999)

Determine Potential Causes of the Problem

1) Determining potential causes requires research. Look at all the data available to you. Talk with your employees and peers, and search out potential causes.
2) Assess the possible causes. Don't jump to conclusions about the solution.
3) Evaluate causes and prioritize them based upon their impact on the problem.

[105.4] 2.15.4 (09-15-1999)

Define Courses of Action To Address Identified Causes: Balance Checking Matrix

1) In this step, you will be brainstorming to identify solutions that will address the most significant causes.
2) Think creatively. Write down all possible solutions. *Remember to include "do nothing" as a potential course of action and evaluate the impact of doing nothing in the Balance Checking Matrix.*
3) Once you have identified possible solutions use the Balance Checking Matrix . . . to consider their impact on all three balanced measures.
4) Remember, the Balance Checking Matrix is not a "decision matrix" in that you should not simply select the alternative with the most pluses. It is intended to ensure that each Balanced Measure area is considered. It also helps identify any Balanced Measure area where you may need to do something else to reduce possible negative impacts.

Courses of Action: Balance Checking Matrix Indicate "+", "–", or "0" impact on measure and provide brief rationale for rating **Form 12302 (7-1999) Cat. No. 28073Z**			
	Impact on Measure		
Proposed Courses of Action (State specific cause being addressed)	**Employee Satisfaction**	**Customer Satisfaction**	**Business Results**
Course of Action 1			
Course of Action 2			
Course of Action 3			

A) When working through the matrix remember: For each alternative, assign a positive, negative, or neutral rating for the impact this alternative might have on each of the three balanced measures:
- Positive impact with "+"
- Negative impact with "–"
- Neutral or no impact with "0"

B) Write out the justification for each rating. This helps to document your reasoning for subsequent evaluation if necessary. For example, if there is a negative impact on employee satisfaction, what is that negative impact?

C) In selecting a course of action:
- Consider how the course of action supports the IRS mission and Strategic Goals.
- Consider which course of action may be the most realistic/least costly to implement.
- Collaborate with others on making the final selection.

[105.4] 2.15.5 (09-15-1999)

Determine a Course of Action

1) Select a course of action that will have the greatest impact on solving the problem in order to best support the IRS mission and strategic goals. Communicate the decision in terms of how it impacts employee satisfaction, customer satisfaction, and business results to ensure understanding that all three balanced measures were considered.

[105.4] 2.15.6 (09-15-1999)

Implement a Course of Action

1) Create a detailed action plan that identifies the steps to be taken in implementing the course of action.

[105.4] 2.15.7 (09-15-1999)

Track Effectiveness of the Course of Action

1) Your action plan should address how you intend to follow up and monitor the effectiveness of the selected course of action. This step reinforces the Review and Revise aspects of the Management Model.

[105.4] 2.16 (09-15-1999)

How Leaders Can Successfully Use the Balanced Measurement System

1) "What you do" speaks more loudly than what you say. There are many actions that can be taken to demonstrate commitment to Balanced Measures and to create a work environment that equally fosters Employee Satisfaction, Customer Satisfaction, and Business Results.

2) The first place to start is to clearly communicate your commitment by using the Balanced Measures approach in all your dealings with customers and employees. When making business decisions, ask "How will this impact customers, employees, and business results?"

3) Overall:
- Be a role model and let others see you using a balanced approach in decision-making.
- Communicate decisions in terms of how the decision impacts employee satisfaction, customer satisfaction, and business results.
- Mentor others. Help them make balanced business decisions, and assist them in developing plans to improve performance.
- Start rewarding, verbally and in writing, those who model the new behavior.
- Be an advocate with upper-level management for the issues outside of your control. Communicate to employees what you have done.
- Roll up your sleeves and get behind the numbers. Get involved.

[105.4] 2.17 (09-15-1999)

Additional Information on the Balanced Measurement System

1) For additional information about the IRS Balanced Measurement System, refer to the Balanced Measures site on the IRS Insider at: www.hq.irs.gov:80/programs/modern/measures/measures.htm.

Exhibit [105.4] 2–1 (09-15-1999). General Questions and Answers about the Balanced Measurement System.

Q1. How do these organizational measures link to individual front-line appraisals?

Individual appraisals of front-line employees will continue to be based on critical elements for their positions. The critical elements in some areas will or have been adjusted to more closely reflect the Service's new priorities as reflected in the Balanced Measures. All employee standards have been updated to reflect the retention standard for all employees that require the "fair and equitable treatment of taxpayers." Overall, evaluations of individual employees must be based on a review of actual work performed as judged against elements and standards and with consideration given to the specific facts and circumstances of each case.

Q2. How do these organizational measures link to individual manager appraisals?

The balanced organizational measures will be inputs to individual manager performance appraisals, but the focus will be on the actions taken to improve performance, not on the numbers. For FY 2000, the critical job elements for managerial employees are being updated to incorporate the balanced measurement system objectives.

Q3. What guarantees are there in the process to prevent managers from relying on "numbers"?

Managers will be expected to look not just at the measurement results but at the facts, circumstances, and specific situations in any area that the measures indicate warrant attention. Managerial expectations have been created to support this change and additional steps to reinforce the new approach include changes to the review processes and the individual performance management processes.

Q4. Will we compare our numerical results against prior years to assess progress?

Measurement results from 1 year will be compared with prior year results to assess progress. This does not mean that a manager's appraisal is determined by how much measures results change over the year. The results can change for numerous reasons, many of which are not under the control of the manager. The actions taken by the manager to improve performance will be what influences the manager's appraisal.

Q5. Why the change?

To better serve taxpayers, we needed to modernize the IRS, including our management practices. The Commissioner has articulated a new vision and mission. This vision focuses on three high-level goals: service to each taxpayer, service to all taxpayers, and productivity through a quality work environment.

Q6. How will we measure Customer Satisfaction?

The Customer Satisfaction measure is based on the customers' perceptions of the service they receive, as obtained through processes such as phone surveys or mail surveys. Survey responses to specific questions will provide the basis for identifying areas with the greatest potential for improvement.

Q7. How will we measure Employee Satisfaction?

There will be two surveys: (1) A Corporate Climate Survey of a sample of IRS employees to check on top level issues and test specific topical issues, e.g., the use of measures, and (2) An Employee Satisfaction Survey available to all IRS employees that will comprise the Employee Satisfaction Score.

Q8. How will we measure Quality in Business Results?

Quality will generally be based on independent review of closed cases or ongoing casework using many of the existing systems, e.g., EQMS—Examination Quality Measurement System, CQMS—Collection Quality Measurement System, CQRS—Centralized Quality Review System.

Q9. How will we measure Quantity in Business Results?

The quantity area of Business Results will consist of outcome neutral measures of production and resource data, such as the number of cases closed or work items completed, as well as a measure of customer outreach efforts.

Q10. When will we have balanced measures for all parts of the IRS?

The development and implementation of balanced measures is [sic] being completed in phases. In Phase I, completed in early 1999, the IRS focused on much of Examination, Collection, and Customer Service. In Phase II, taking place throughout 1999, the focus is on those components of the modernized IRS that are scheduled to roll-out first. In Phase III, which will get underway in late 1999 and early 2000, the remaining components not worked in Phases I & II will be addressed. Until balanced measures are developed across all parts of the IRS, managers and employees can continue to use existing performance measures as appropriate and keeping in mind the overall balanced approach set forth in this chapter.

Exhibit [105.4] 2–2 (09-15-1999). Glossary of Terms.

ACTION PLANS

Specific tactics/actions identified in each work unit, below the division level, to achieve and support the IRS' Business Plans and Operations Plans.

BALANCED MEASURES

Indicator of results for two or more measures considered of equal importance.

BUSINESS PLANS

Identifies major actions to be taken by a Region, Executive Officer for Service Center Operations (EOSCO), Chief, Customer Service Field Operations (CCSFO), District or Service Center in support/ implementation of the Operations Plan and Strategic Goals.

BUSINESS RESULTS MEASURES

Indicators of the quality and quantity of work performed.

CUSTOMER

Any internal or external person or entity to whom you provide services.

CUSTOMER SATISFACTION MEASURE

An indicator of the level of overall satisfaction with service provided by the IRS as perceived by internal or external customers.

DIAGNOSTIC TOOLS

Indicators that are not designated as "Balanced Measures." They are used to discover the factors impacting changes in the Balanced Measures.

EMPLOYEE SATISFACTION MEASURE

An indicator of the level of overall satisfaction with the work environment as perceived by employees.

GOAL

A desired performance objective can be qualitative or quantitative (numeric).

IRS BALANCED MEASURES

Indicators of organizational performance for Customer Satisfaction, Employee Satisfaction, and Business Results.

OPERATIONS PLAN

A high level plan developed annually by the Chief Operations Officer and the Assistant Commissioners. It defines the priorities and identifies the actions that each Assistant Commissioner area will focus on for the upcoming year. The Operations Plan is the focus for the development of Business Plans and Action Plans.

ORGANIZATIONAL MEASURES

Indicators of the progress the IRS is making in achieving its strategic goals and mission.

OUTCOME NEUTRAL

Production or resource data that does not contain information regarding the tax enforcement result reached in any case, e.g., number of cases closed, level of service provided, assistance, and outreach efforts undertaken.

PERFORMANCE MEASURE

An indicator of results for an activity, process, organization, or program.

PERFORMANCE MEASURES RESULT

Numeric outcome of a measure for an activity, process, organization, or program.

QUALITY MEASURE

A numeric indicator of the extent to which completed work meets prescribed standards.

QUANTITY MEASURE

An indicator of outreach efforts, outcome neutral productivity, and resource utilization.

STAKEHOLDERS

Groups or individuals who have a vested interest in an organization. They can be internal or external to IRS.

STRATEGIC GOAL

A strategic goal defines how an organization will carry out its mission over a period. It is expressed in a manner that allows a future assessment to be made on whether the goal was or is being achieved. The goal may be of a programmatic, policy, or management nature.

Exhibit [105.4] 2–3 (09-15-1999). Balanced Measures for Examination, Collection, and Customer Service.

	Customer Satisfaction	Employee Satisfaction	Business Results	
Quality	Quantity* (Volume/Mix)			
Examination Measures	Examination transaction survey score	Examination employee satisfaction survey score	EQMS score % Cases overage	Number of returns closed (by audit category) –Individual < $100K –Individual > $100K –Individual with schedule C or F –Business < $10 M –Business > $10 M Time spent on outreach (work in progress)

Quality	Customer Satisfaction Quantity* (Volume/Mix)	Employee Satisfaction	Business Results	
Collection Measures	Collection transaction survey score	Collection employee satisfaction score	CQMS Score % Cases overage % Offers in compromise processed within 6 months	Number of cases closed –TDA –TDI Time spent on outreach (work in progress)
Customer Service Measures	Toll Free –Transaction survey score	Toll Free –Employee satisfaction survey score	Toll Free –Quality (Tax Law and Accounts) –Timeliness	Toll Free –Level of service –Adherence to scheduled hours –Time spent on education/outreach (work in progress)
	ACS –Transaction survey score	ACS –Employee satisfaction survey score	ACS –Quality –Timeliness –Customer relations –Overage inventory	ACS –Level of service –Time spent on outreach (work in progress)
	Service Center Exam –Transaction survey score	Service Center Exam –Employee satisfaction survey score	Service Center Exam –Exam/ASFR Quality –Overage inventory	Service Center Exam –Exam/ASFR closures –Time spent on outreach (work in progress)

ORGANIZATIONAL PERFORMANCE MANAGEMENT AND THE IRS BALANCED MEASUREMENT SYSTEM

The material that follows is adapted from the Office of Organizational Performance Management, Internal Revenue Service, Department of the Treasury, *Organizational Performance Management and the IRS Balanced Measurement System,* June 2000, Publication 3561 (Rev. 6-2000), Catalog Number 28908N. It can be accessed on the IRS Web site (www.irs.gov/prod/news/measures.html).

The IRS will use balanced measures, comprised of both output and outcome measures[1], at both the strategic level and the operational level to measure organizational performance. At the individual level, critical elements and critical performance expectations that support and align with the IRS mission and balanced measures approach will be the basis by which employees are evaluated.

In September 1999, a Balanced Measures Regulation was issued to formally establish the IRS new performance management system. The issuance of the regulation, which followed a public comment period, sets forth the structure for measuring organizational and employee performance within the IRS. A copy of the regulation is available on the IRS Insider and the IRS Digital Daily (www.irs.gov).

At the strategic level, measures will be used to assess overall performance in delivering on the mission and three strategic goals. Strategic measures will apply to the organization as a whole and to each of the major operating and functional divisions in the modernized IRS.

At the operational management level, balanced measures are used to assess the effectiveness of program and service delivery of particular components of the organization.

The IRS has translated its mission into three strategic goals of service to each taxpayer, service to all taxpayers,

---

[1] Output measures reflect units produced or services produced by a program, e.g., cases closed, calls answered. Outcome measures reflect results — the changes or accomplishments that are achieved, e.g., customer satisfaction, employee satisfaction, quality.

ORGANIZATIONAL PERFORMANCE MANAGEMENT AND THE IRS BALANCED MEASUREMENT SYSTEM

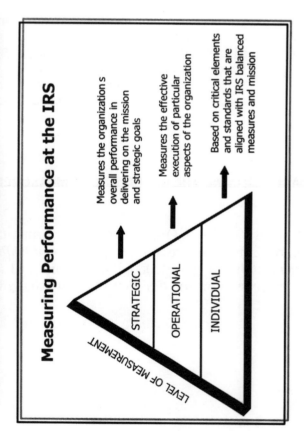

Measuring Performance at the IRS

STRATEGIC — Measures the organization's overall performance in delivering on the mission and strategic goals

OPERATIONAL — Measures the effective execution of particular aspects of the organization

INDIVIDUAL — Based on critical elements and standards that are aligned with IRS balanced measures and mission

LEVEL OF MEASUREMENT

The IRS Balanced Measurement System has been developed as part of the effort to modernize the IRS and to reflect the Service's priorities, as articulated in the IRS mission. This new approach to measurement is intended to help shift the focus of individuals and the organization away from achieving a specific target or number to achieving the overall mission and strategic goals of the IRS.

To help ensure balance, each of the three components of balanced measures customer satisfaction, employee satisfaction, and business results will be carefully considered by the IRS when setting organizational objectives, establishing goals, assessing progress and results, and evaluating individual performance.

and productivity through a quality work environment. These three strategic goals are supported by the balanced measures as depicted in the next table. This framework will assist the IRS in describing how programs and initiatives tie to achievement of the mission and goals as reflected in improvements in the measurement results.

Relationship of Strategic Goals to Balanced Measures

STRATEGIC GOAL	BALANCED MEASURE
• Objectives	
Service to Each Taxpayer • Make filing easier • Provide first quality service to each taxpayer needing assistance • Provide prompt, professional, helpful treatment to taxpayers in cases where additional taxes may be due	Customer Satisfaction
Service to All Taxpayers • Increase Fairness of Compliance • Increase Overall Compliance	Business Results (Quality, Quantity & Outreach)
Productivity through a Quality Work Environment • Increase employee job satisfaction • Hold agency employment stable while economy grows and service improves	Employee Satisfaction

OPERATIONAL LEVEL BALANCED MEASURES FRAMEWORK

Service to Each Taxpayer/Customer Satisfaction

The service to each taxpayer goal is measured from the customer's point of view. The goal of the Customer Satisfaction element is to provide accurate and professional services to internal and external customers in a courteous, timely manner. The customer satisfaction goals and accomplishments of operating units within the IRS are determined on the basis of customer feedback collected via methods such as questionnaires, surveys and other types of information gathering mechanisms. Information to measure customer satisfaction for a particular work unit is gathered from a sample of the customers served. Customers are permitted to provide information requested for these purposes anonymously. Customers may include individual taxpayers, organizational units or employees within the IRS and external groups affected by the services performed by the IRS operating unit.

Service to All Taxpayers / Business Results

The service to all taxpayers goal is gauged through a combination of quality, quantity and outreach measures. The goal of the Business Results elements is to generate a productive quantity of work in a quality manner and to provide meaningful outreach to all customers. The business results measures consist of numerical scores determined under the elements of Quantity and Quality.

♦ The quantity measures, which are to be used in conjunction with the quality, customer satisfaction, and employee satisfaction measures[2], provide information about the volume and mix of work products and services produced by IRS operating units and consist of outcome-neutral production and resource data. Examples include the number of cases closed, work items completed, customer education, assistance and outreach efforts undertaken, hours expended and similar inventory, workload and staffing information.

---

[2] The Balanced Measures Regulation restricts the use of quantity measures for organizational units with employees who exercise judgement with regard to enforcement of the tax law. Quantity measures may be used to set organizational goals or to evaluate organizational performance in these areas only if done in conjunction with the other elements of the Balanced Measurement System. (See section 801.2(b) of the Regulation.)

◆ The quality measures provide information about how well IRS operating units developed and delivered their products and services. The quality measures are determined based upon a comparison of a sample of work items handled by certain functions or organizational units against a prescribed set of standards that incorporate the customers point of view. Additional quality measures will gauge the accuracy and timeliness of the products and services provided.

Productivity Through a Quality Work Environment / Employee Satisfaction

The productivity through a quality work environment goal is assessed via measures of employee satisfaction. The goal of the Employee Satisfaction element is to create an enabling work environment for employees by providing quality leadership, adequate training, and effective support services. The employee satisfaction ratings to be given within the IRS are determined on the basis of information gathered via survey. All employees have an opportunity to provide information regarding employee satisfaction under conditions that guarantee them anonymity.

ADDITIONAL LINKAGES BETWEEN BALANCED MEASURES AND STRATEGIC GOALS

The relationship of operational performance measures to strategic goals as described above is intended to help illustrate the primary linkages between the measures and goals. The IRS recognizes that secondary linkages between the measures and the three goals also exist. For example, efforts to improve employee satisfaction in support of the *productivity through a quality work environment* goal

often result in improvements to customer service thereby enhancing the *service to each taxpayer* goal. Similarly, quality efforts that improve the timeliness and accuracy of work performed not only result in improved business results and *service to all taxpayers* but can also result in improved levels of customer satisfaction and better *service to each taxpayer*.

USE OF ENFORCEMENT DATA

In addition to the balanced measures, the IRS collects a great deal of other information about programs and services that is useful for purposes of tracking, analyzing and reflecting the factors that affect overall performance. Some of this information, such as dollars collected, dollars assessed, liens filed, and seizures executed, are *records of*

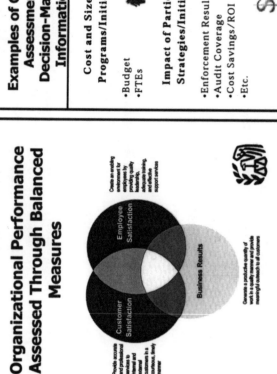

Organizational Performance Assessed Through Balanced Measures

Performance Assessment Framework

Employee Satisfaction — Create an enabling environment for employees by providing quality leadership, adequate training, and effective support services

Customer Satisfaction — Provide accurate and professional services to internal and external customers in a courteous, timely manner

Business Results — Generate a productive quantity of work in a quality manner and provide meaningful outreach to all customers

Examples of Other Assessment, Decision-Making Information

Cost and Size of Programs/Initiatives
•Budget
•FTEs

Impact of Particular Strategies/Initiatives
•Enforcement Results
•Audit Coverage
•Cost Savings/ROI
•Etc.

tax enforcement results which the organization is prohibited by law from using to evaluate or to impose or suggest production quotas or goals for any employee.

Therefore, in the IRS Balanced Measurement System, enforcement statistics are not measures of performance at either the operational or strategic level. Enforcement statistics are used, however, at a strategic level to make projections for and to assess the effectiveness of particular strategies and initiatives. Such information is intended to help illustrate the potential impact of resource and strategy decisions on factors that affect overall compliance, such as audit coverage.

DEVELOPING BALANCED MEASURES

At the Strategic Level

As described earlier, measures at the strategic level are meaningful for the service as a whole and for each of the operating and functional divisions. They will be comprised of measures such as burden, compliance, overall customer satisfaction and employee satisfaction, and productivity. Taxpayer burden and voluntary compliance, for example, are among the most important outcomes affected by IRS activities for which measurements at the strategic level are critical but also inherently difficult to develop. The challenge is in identifying valid and reliable ways to measure them.

To date, the balanced measures effort has focused primarily on the development of measures at the operational level. However, work began in FY 1999 and

will accelerate in FY 2000 to develop strategic measures for roll-out in the modernized IRS during FY 2001. Once fully implemented, strategic measures will be used by the IRS in its annual performance plan at the Strategic Management Level and for each Operating Division and Functional Division.

At the Operational Level

The IRS is utilizing a four-step process for the development of balanced measures in each of its Operating Divisions and Functional Divisions. The total duration from start to finish of this process varies depending on the availability and usability of existing measures as well as the complexity and related system requirements of the final set of measures selected.

In Phase I, Conceptualization and Problem Definition, the measures team is convened, a charter and timeline is

Balanced Measures Development Process

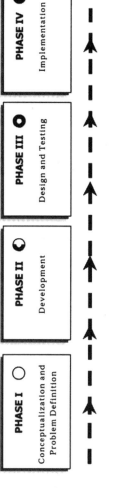

prepared, and a baseline of current measures, if applicable, is completed. The teams are comprised of national office and field IRS personnel and union representatives. In Phase II, Development, the team identifies a proposed set of measures for each element of the balanced measurement framework customer satisfaction, employee satisfaction, and business results. During this phase, best practice

5

reviews are conducted and a pro/con analysis is applied to each proposed measure. Phase II concludes upon approval of the proposed set of measures by the IRS Organizational Performance Management Steering Committee. For purposes of obtaining additional feedback on the proposed measures, information is also shared with external stakeholders and others via press releases and the IRS Digital Daily web site. In Phase III, Design and Testing, the approved measures are thoroughly tested and revised as necessary. An implementation plan is prepared for the final phase, Implementation. During implementation Phase IV, any management information system requirements and cost and personnel needs are resolved. Prior to rolling out the measures, a communication and training plan is completed and ownership of the measures is clearly established in the relevant Operating or Functional Division.

PROGRESS UPDATE

The IRS completed balanced measures development for the Examination, Collection and three Customer Service product lines in calendar year (CY) 1998. In CY 1999, additional balanced measures were approved for Tax Exempt and Government Entities[3], Large and Mid-Size Business, Appeals, Taxpayer Advocate Service, Research, Statistics of Income, and additional Customer Service product lines. These measures are undergoing final design and implementation. Other measures teams underway in CY 1999 that are expected to have approved balanced measures in early CY 2000 include Information Systems, Criminal Investigation, Submission Processing, and Agency Wide Shared Services. All remaining areas, including Small Business/Self-Employed and the Wage & Investment Operating Divisions, will commence measures development in CY 2000. For the Small Business/Self Employed and Wage and Investment Operating Divisions, much of the balanced measures work that has already been completed for the Examination, Collection, and Customer Service functions will be applicable. The Measures Development Progress table reports on progress for the Operating Divisions and Functional Divisions.

Measures Development Progress

Large and Mid-Size Business	● ●
Tax Exempt and Government Entities	● ●
Small Business and Self Employed*	○
Wage and Investment*	○
Information Systems	◐ ◐
Agency-Wide Shared Services	◐ ◐
Taxpayer Advocate Service	●
Criminal Investigation	◐ ◐
Appeals	● ●
Counsel	◐ ◐
CORE	◐ ◐

KEY:
○ Not yet started or Phase I
◑ Phase II, Development Underway
◕ Phase III, Testing and Final Development
● Phase IV, Implementation   As of 12/99

*Much of the balanced measures development work already completed in Examination, Collection and Customer Service will be transferable and applicable to these Operating Divisions.

[3] Balanced measures were approved for most of the Tax Exempt portion of TE/GE. Additional measures work is yet to be done for the Coordinated Exam Program, Customer Account Services, and Government Entities.

The transition from the old ways of doing business to the new, modernized IRS will take time. The measures reflected in this document will help move the IRS in that direction and bring the organization a step closer to a truly balanced framework of measurements at the strategic and operational levels.

As the balanced measures are tested and used throughout the organization, lessons will be learned and refinements in the measures may be necessary. However, the basic concept of what needs to be measured — customer satisfaction, employee satisfaction, and business results — will remain stable and firmly grounded in the organizational design principles of the modernized IRS.

SUMMARY

In moving forward with the creation of a new organization focused on providing America's taxpayers top quality service by helping them understand and meet their tax responsibilities and by applying the tax law with integrity and fairness to all, it is essential that the IRS change how it measures organizational performance. Key to this change is the development of new, balanced measures that are aligned with the mission and strategic goals of the new IRS.

CHAPTER 7
Systems Executive Officer for Manpower and Personnel: Strategic Direction and Performance Measurement

During the past several years, one of the most interesting applications of the Balanced Scorecard has been in a Navy program office in New Orleans, Louisiana. Until the past year, the office was in the Naval Reserve Headquarters (HQ) in New Orleans. In the past year, the office has had a name change to Navy Program Executive Office for Information Technology (PEO/IT). The office now reports to the Navy Secretariat in Washington, D.C.

This is an interesting application of the Balanced Scorecard. For the past several years, the program office has been developing its performance blueprint, with strong management support, with four goals: (1) people, (2) customer, (3) business, and (4) technical. These areas are generally consistent with those of Kaplan and Norton.[1] Figure 7–1 is adapted from the Draft Systems Executive Officer for Manpower and Personnel (SEO/MP) Strategic Direction dated July 22, 1999. The strategic direction is aligned with two objectives under each goal and five to ten performance measures aligned under each objective. There are a total of 49 performance measures listed.

The update for Fiscal Year (FY) 2000 is adapted from the PEO(IT) Information Technology Center (ITC) Strategic Direction FY 2000–2005 (Figure 7–2). The mission and vision have some changes, but the four goals are the same. There are also several changes in the objectives.

Figure 7–3, adapted from the ITC Performance Blueprint FY 2000, retains the four strategic goals and list eight annual goals for FY 2000. The performance measures are reduced from 49 to 36 and aligned with the short-term strategies supporting eight annual goals and then supporting the four long-term strategic goals.

---

[1]Kaplan, Robert S., and David P. Norton. *The Balanced Scorecard.* Boston: Harvard Business School Press, 1996.

Figure 7–1

SEO/MP Strategic Direction

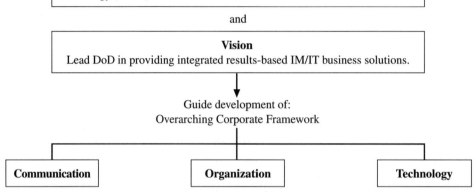

Mission
Improve the Department of Defense (DoD) readiness and operational capability by delivering effective, efficient integrated information management/information technology (IM/IT) solutions.

and

Vision
Lead DoD in providing integrated results-based IM/IT business solutions.

Guide development of:
Overarching Corporate Framework

| **Communication** | **Organization** | **Technology** |

Strategic Direction—Leads to Goal Development

Goal 1: People Goal

Establish an efficient and effective organizational infrastructure and a results-oriented workforce.

Objectives

Objective 1.1:	**Objective 1.2:**
Develop and establish an organizational infrastructure that supports efficient and effective use of the workforce.	Develop a workforce with the skills, core values, and attributes required to effectively manage and support the acquisition/IT process.

Strategies

Establish a premier Information Technology Center that leverages the exchange of ideas, information, research, and development.	Develop near-, short-, and long-term total workforce requirements.
Define and implement the organizational structure.	Align total workforce requirements with recruiting, training, and retention programs/processes to maintain consistency with industry best practices.
Define or develop and document the organization's work processes.	
Define core competencies and assess abilities of the current workforce to support the organizational mission.	Partner with local and state universities and private sector firms to develop and acquire interns and team members.
Develop individual training plans that support workforce gaps.	Conduct transition orientation to instill core values and work ethics.
Develop internal communications program.	Institute employee recognition and reward program.

Performance Measures

Establish premier Information Technology Center by TBD.	Identify and develop total workforce requirements by TBD.
Complete organization stand-up by TBD.	Conduct semiannual analysis to ensure alignment of human resource processes with total workforce requirements.
Establish and implement an enterprise-level data repository and architecture.	
Consolidate and collate work processes into a process management tool by TBD.	Increase number of formal partnerships with local and state universities and private sector firms for personnel asset development and retention by TBD percent.
Complete internal strengths, weaknesses, opportunities, and threats (SWOT) analysis by TBD.	Ensure all employees receive orientation training no later than TBD.
Complete ongoing skills assessment by TBD and institute semiannual skills assessment process by TBD.	Conduct 360-degree survey to validate orientation training.
Develop internal communications process by TBD.	Baseline employee satisfaction.
Conduct quarterly focus group to measure effectiveness of internal communications program.	Stand up Employee Incentive Program by TBD.

Goal 2: Customer Goal

Consistently meet customer requirements and exceed customer expectations.

Objectives

Objective 2.1:

Develop a program that identifies customer expectations and requirements.

Objective 2.2:

Increase customer satisfaction

Strategies

Baseline customer expectations and requirements.

Monitor customer expectations and requirements to ensure services provided meet or exceed customer needs.

Provide a feedback mechanism for customers to ensure evolving requirements are addressed in a timely manner.

Become a full participating member in the requirements generation process.

Establish a program that measures the effectiveness of the organization's ability to meet customer expectations and requirements.

Conduct one-on-one interviews, focus groups, and surveys to identify the level of customer satisfaction.

Performance Measures

Complete customer expectations and requirements baseline by TBD.

Establish program that monitors customer expectations and requirements to ensure services provided meet or exceed customer needs by TBD.

Develop a feedback mechanism to ensure evolving requirements are addressed in a timely manner by TBD.

Begin participation in customer requirements generation process by TBD.

Develop internal policies, processes, and procedures that support the program to measure the organization's ability to meet customer expectations and requirements by TBD.

Establish internal process that facilitates one-on-one interviews, focus groups, and surveys to identify the level of customer satisfaction by TBD.

Goal 3: Business Goal

Improve long-term business performance through implementation of repeatable best business processes and practices.

Objectives

Objective 3.1:

Benchmark successful corporate/federal best practices.

Objective 3.2:

Enable business/IT management improvement.

Strategies

Become a member of the Federal Benchmarking Consortium and/or similar organizations.

Assess applicable benchmarking studies and establish pilot program(s) that leverage best process improvements.

Investigate best corporate management processes.

Establish a training program in benchmarking study development.

Establish strategic management program.

Institute business process management program.

Leverage commercial IM/IT best business practices.

Benchmark successful government/business IT management initiatives.

Establish an IT capital planning and investment control process.

Facilitate business process reengineering (BPR) to increase degree of fit between functional requirements and existing technology.

Establish a vehicle for storage, categorization, and retrieval of corporate intellectual properties.

Performance Measures

Gain membership to Federal Benchmarking Consortium and/or similar organizations by TBD.

Establish appropriate pilot programs that leverage best process improvements.

Ensure management processes are aligned with federal/commercial guidance.

Establish a training program in benchmarking study development by TBD.

Implement strategic management program by TBD.

Develop an operational framework for each functional level office by TBD.

Institute business process management program and tool by TBD.

Maintain membership in one or more IM/IT best practice repositories.

Establish and implement a benchmarking study program/process by TBD.

Establish Investment Control Board by TBD.

Establish management process and tools necessary to support capital planning and investment control process by TBD.

Establish baseline of existing IT portfolio by TBD.

Facilitate BPR studies prior to investigating COTS/GOTS/new technology solutions.

Establish a Knowledge Management Center by TBD.

Goal 4: Technical Goal

> Delivery and sustain integrated enterprise IM/IT solutions.

Objectives

Objective 4.1:	Objective 4.2:
Develop and establish the methodologies, policies, processes, and procedures to deliver and sustain integrated enterprise IM/IT solutions.	Fully leverage COTS/GOTS technology prior to developing new IM/IT solutions.

Strategies

Provide an integrated results-based enterprise strategy for delivering and sustaining IM/IT solutions.	Establish a program to research and prove out new products and emerging technologies.
Ensure compliance with DoD, GAO, and OMB IT management requirements.	Populate Knowledge Management Center with IM/IT trade-off analyses.
Establish Joint Requirements Group to perform trade-off analyses of proposed technical solutions.	Use COTS/GOTS product where applicable and feasible.
Ensure that technical/functional architectures align with federal guidelines.	Establish performance management process/program office to assess how well solutions meet requirements.
Provide a process to customize COTS/GOTS applications for assembly into reusable solutions.	
Establish a world-class Systems Management Center to deliver IM/IT services.	

Performance Measures

Develop the enterprise strategy to deliver and sustain IM/IT solutions by TBD.	Stand up research program by TBD.
Establish a process to audit enterprise IT management strategies to ensure outputs and outcomes are aligned with desired results by TBD.	Begin populating Knowledge Management Center by TBD.
	Complete a COTS/GOTS business case for each proposed solution by TBD.
Establish Joint Requirements Group by TBD.	Complete a Conference Room Pilot for each proposed COTS/GOTS solution by TBD.
Document degree of fit between technical solutions and requirements.	Establish performance management process/program office by TBD.
Provide documented analyses to the Knowledge Management Center for reuse.	
Establish process to audit architectures for alignment by TBD.	
Develop and establish an information security program by TBD.	
Establish process framework to customize COTS/GOTS applications for assembly into reusable solutions by TBD.	
Stand up Systems Management Center by TBD.	

Source: Adapted from Systems Executive Officer for Manpower and Personnel, New Orleans, Louisiana, July 22, 1999. Draft—22 July 1999. Revised Team Proposal 5.

Figure 7–2

PEO(IT) ITC Strategic Direction FY 2000–2005

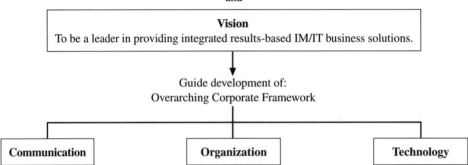

Mission
To improve the Department of Defense (DoD) readiness and organizational capability by delivering effective enterprise-wide integrated information management/information technology solutions and life cycle support that reduces the cost of supported functions.

and

Vision
To be a leader in providing integrated results-based IM/IT business solutions.

Guide development of:
Overarching Corporate Framework

| Communication | Organization | Technology |

Goal 1: People Goal

Establish an efficient and effective organizational infrastructure and a results-oriented workforce.

Objectives

Objective 1.1:	Objective 1.2:
Continue establishing an organizational infrastructure that supports the efficient and effective use of the workforce.	Sustain a continually improving workforce with the skills, competencies, and attributes required to effectively manage and support the acquisition/IT process.

Long-term Strategies

Sustain development of an enterprise solutions center that leverages the exchange of ideas, information, research, and development.	Build workforce that can be effective and flexible in assimilating emerging technologies.
Align infrastructure and competencies with PEO(IT) superior and piece organizations.	Develop initiatives that will produce a sustainable workforce that will either allow for growth or replacement.
Develop a comprehensive communications program.	Mitigate workforce risk through continual assessment of: • Personnel availability • Skills • Associated costs.
Plan for growth.	Provide a learning environment that enhances change and is a fun place to work.

Goal 2: Customer Goal

Consistently meet customer requirements and exceed customer expectations.

Objectives

Objective 2.1:

Design, develop, and deploy a multitiered Customer Relationship Management program built on best federal commercial practices.

Objective 2.2:

Serve fundamental customer needs with unprecedented levels of performance while generating cost savings.

Long-term Strategies

Mature a process to identify, document, and manage customer requirements and expectations.

Implement and sustain a Customer Relationship Management program.

Never stop improving customer services, the business model, processes, and performance.

Institutionalize the Customer Relationship Management paradigm at all organizational levels.

Sustain outcome-oriented feedback mechanisms to ensure service levels are addressed in a timely manner.

Maximize reusability of our competencies to:
• Decrease our time to market.
• Reduce our costs.
• Reduce our risk.
• Improve our quality.
• Delight our customers.

Goal 3: Business Goal

Improve long-term business performance through implementation of repeatable best business processes and practices.

Objectives

Objective 3.1:

Establish and replicate the IT business model to identify and facilitate process improvement and re-engineering opportunities.

Objective 3.2:

Enable business performance improvement throughout the organization.

Long-term Strategies

Benchmark, document, and adapt successful corporate/government best business practices.

Identify, baseline, and document organizational processes.

Align the organization's business and management processes with federal reform guidelines, current legislation, and industry-recognized commercial standards.

Facilitate replication by establishing a business framework that supports knowledge transfer and by fostering a culture change to leverage its utility.

Refine the results-driven Strategic/Performance Management program.

Institutionalize a Performance Management system to measure the effectiveness of organizational processes and use the information to improve effectiveness and efficiency.

Leverage organizational learning best practices.

Provide requisite training needed to leverage performance management.

Embrace the Actions Collaboration Team (ACT) philosophy to improve business performance.

Goal 4: Technical Goal

Deliver and sustain integrated enterprise IM/IT solutions.

Objectives

Objective 4.1:	Objective 4.2:
Build and sustain a technical infrastructure/architecture that will allow cost-efficient cross-functional support.	Improve technical solutions delivery and support.

Long-term Strategies

Refine and deploy repeatable acquisition and development processes.	Develop initiatives that will foster collaborative research and development efforts.
Identify, implement, and maintain flexible evolutionary architectures.	Leverage COTS/GOTS technology.
Sustain world-class technology management, delivery, and support systems.	Manage solution integration and support delivery to PMs.
Focus, simplify, and standardize on all fronts of technical infrastructure and architecture.	Assess how well solutions and support meet requirements through the Performance Management program.

Source: Adapted from Program Executive Office for Information Technology, New Orleans, Louisiana, February 4, 2000.

Figure 7–3

ITC Performance Blueprint FY 2000
Multiyear Strategic Direction

Mission

To improve the Department of Defense (DoD) readiness and organizational capability by delivering effective enterprise-wide integrated information management/information technology solutions and life cycle support that reduces the cost of supported functions.

Vision

To be a leader in providing integrated results-based IM/IT business solutions.

People Goal

Strategic Goal:
Establish an efficient and effective organizational infrastructure and a results-oriented workforce.

Annual Goal 1	**Annual Goal 2**
Establish an organizational infrastructure that provides the foundation for accomplishing our mission and vision.	Retain/hire the requisite employees to lay the foundation for a results-oriented workforce.

Short-term Strategies

Complete the development and stand-up of the organizational infrastructure.	Baseline and improve employee satisfaction.
Align infrastructure and competencies with PEC(IT) superior and peer organizations.	Develop initiatives that will foster creativity and innovation and increase retention rates.
Utilize the Communications program to assist with institutionalizing the infrastructure.	Develop mitigation strategies to minimize risks associated with a ready pool of trained, qualified IT professionals.

Action Items

Define the organizational structure.	Identify total workforce requirements and gaps.
Assign organizational roles and responsibilities.	Partner with academia to design programs that will cultivate qualified IT professionals.
Charter an ACT to assist with the organizational stand-up.	Develop departmental training programs.
Develop and document departmental competencies.	Design individual, team, and departmental reward and recognition programs.
Write an internal/external Communications Plan.	
Develop a communications schedule and implementation plan.	Initiate a personnel risk mitigation program to address skills assessment, personnel availability, and associated labor costs.

Customer

> **Strategic Goal:**
> Consistently meet customer requirements and exceed customer expectations.

Annual Goal 3	**Annual Goal 4**
Design and develop a multitiered Customer Relationship Management (CRM) program built on best federal/commercial practices.	Ready the organization for successful deployment of the CRM program.

Short-term Strategies

Define and mature a process to identify, document, and manage customer requirements and expectations.	Educate all members of the organization about the value of CRM and their individual responsibilities in ensuring program success.
Develop and implement a prototype CRM process and measure its effectiveness.	Define the relationship among customers/stakeholders and the enterprise.

Action Items

Charter a customer-focus task force to handle near-term CRM initiatives.	Develop an educational/training program to institutionalize CRM across the enterprise.
Develop tier-specific CRM tasks.	Define external CRM organizational roles and responsibilities.
Define internal CRM organizational roles and responsibilities.	
Charter an ACT to develop the CRM program.	
Develop the CRM measurement methodology.	
Implement the prototype.	
Measure, document, and report prototype CRM results.	

Business

> **Strategic Goal:**
> Improve long-term business performance through implementation of repeatable best business processes and practices.

Annual Goal 5	**Annual Goal 6**
Develop a methodology to identify and facilitate process improvement and re-engineering opportunities.	Initiate business performance improvement throughout the organization.

Short-term Strategies

Identify, baseline, and document selected organizational processes.	Provide performance management training based on best industry/government practices.
Standardize a methodology to maximize repeatability of processes throughout the enterprise.	Stand up ACTs and identify their responsibilities in improving business performance.

Action Items

Establish/charter an Enterprise Process Management team.	Define training requirements.
Select a suite of tools and identify applicable process standards to accomplish the process management tasks.	Develop training plans and identify resources.
Pilot a process management initiative, measure the results, and adjust the initiative accordingly.	Train key personnel.
Benchmark similar process management efforts and adjust the methodology.	Develop guidelines for the use, chartering, and resourcing of ACTs.
Continue development of the enterprise process management repository.	

Technical

Strategic Goal:
Deliver and sustain integrated enterprise IM/IT solutions.

Annual Goal 7	**Annual Goal 8**
Build a technical infrastructure/architecture that allows for cross-functional support.	Improve technical solutions delivery and support.

Short-term Strategies

Develop and deploy repeatable ITC acquisition models/processes.	Leverage research and development partnerships to investigate leading edge best-of-class methods of improving technical solutions delivery and support.
Define the enterprise architecture approach.	
Develop and deploy the enterprise technical architecture.	Institutionalize a process to use COTS/GOTS technology.

Action Items

Develop and deploy the ITC pre-Milestone acquisition process.	Expand partnerships from pure academic relationships to those that foster research and development.
Develop and deploy the ITC workflow process.	
Develop the enterprise operational, systems, and technical architecture processes.	Pilot the use of a COTS/GOTS selection process.
	Adapt the COTS/GOTS selection process and standardize its use within the ITC.
Design and implement the enterprise technical architecture.	

Source: Adapted from Program Executive Office for Information Technology, New Orleans, Louisiana, February 4, 2000.

CHAPTER 8

A Report on Managing Performance in the Government

The Interagency Work Group on Performance Management reported out in February 2000 with a 17-page report entitled *Report to the President's Management Council on Managing Performance in the Government*. The report contained three major themes: (1) expect excellence, (2) establish accountability, and (3) take timely action. The report, which is comprehensive, identifies opportunities and challenges for each theme as well as action recommendations. They include many GPRA issues. Comments indicate that agencies that are using Balanced Measures are achieving real breakthroughs in how they plan and communicate expectations.

INTERAGENCY WORK GROUP ON PERFORMANCE MANAGEMENT

The following material is adapted from the Interagency Work Group on Performance Management, *Report to the President's Management Council on Managing Performance in the Government*, Washington, D.C., National Partnership for Reinventing Government, February 2000.

Table of Contents

Message to the President's Management Council
Premises and Principles
Themes
  Theme 1: Expect Excellence
    Communicate Expectations
      Recommendations
    Create a Climate for Excellence
      Recommendations
  Theme 2: Establish Accountability
    Hold Supervisors Accountable for Managing Performance
      Recommendations
    Include Performance Management Outcomes in HR Accountability Systems
      Recommendations
  Theme 3: Take Timely Action
    Intervene Early
      Recommendations
    Support Supervisors Taking Performance-Based Actions
      Recommendations

Appendices
A. Summary of Recommendations
    Theme 1: Expect Excellence
    Theme 2: Establish Accountability
    Theme 3: Take Timely Action
B. Agency Innovations and Resources
    Theme 1: Expect Excellence
        Communicate Expectations
        Create a Climate for Excellence
    Theme 2: Establish Accountability
        Hold Supervisors Accountable for Managing Performance
    Include Performance Management Outcomes in HR Accountability
    Systems
    Theme 3: Take Timely Action
        Intervene Early
        Support Supervisors Taking Performance-Based Actions

This report is available for downloading as a PDF document.

Message to the President's Management Council

We are pleased to present this Report to the President's Management Council on Managing Performance in the Government. This is in response to your mandate for actions and recommendations to address the issue of employee performance management.

Our work group of human resources management executives concluded that a report that could be shared with all federal agencies would demonstrate top-level commitment to excellent performance. The inclusion of concrete recommendations and information on best practices provides practical assistance for achieving excellence throughout the federal government.

Paul D. Barnes
Social Security Administration

Carolyn Cohen
Department of the Interior

Tim Dirks
Department of Energy

Kay Frances Dolan
Department of the Treasury

Sharlyn A. Grigsby
Department of State

Carol Harvey
National Partnership for
Reinventing Government

Vicki A. Novak
National Aeronautics and Space Administration

Evelyn M. White
Department of Health and Human Services

Henry Romero
Office of Personnel Management

Steve Cohen
Office of Personnel Management

Joyce Edwards
Office of Personnel Management

Premises and Principles

- The federal workforce is comprised of dedicated, hardworking public servants who strive to deliver value to Americans.
- As a result, Americans can expect performance excellence when the workforce is engaged and involved in designing a results-oriented, performance-based, and customer-focused system that delivers that value.
- Federal leaders and managers create a climate for excellence by communicating their vision, values, and expectations clearly, and by:
  - creating an environment for continual learning;
  - working in partnership with employees to ensure they reach their full potential;
  - recognizing and rewarding excellence with financial incentives and non-financial incentives, such as increased flexibility to do jobs, more meaningful work, and achieving a sense of accomplishment; and
  - taking timely action to both reward and correct performance appropriately, ensuring that excellence is the standard for all.
- Feedback from customers and employees, along with operations results, will be the basis for credible and useful performance evaluations. Employees are personally responsible for being results-oriented, performance-based, and customer-focused, and for providing feedback that holds their leaders, managers, and colleagues accountable for achieving excellence.
- Leaders and managers will work in partnership with unions to promote constructive discussion about all aspects of performance management, including improving employee performance.
- Leaders, managers, and employees have a mutual obligation to provide value and excellence to America. This requires each individual to be continually challenged to perform their best. Taking action to improve the performance of each individual is imperative to achieving agencies' missions.
- The President's Management Council—indeed the entire Administration—is committed to pursuing effective performance management throughout government.

These premises and principles are reflected in **three major themes**. For each theme, this report identifies opportunities and challenges, offers substantiating evidence where appropriate, and makes recommendations for action.

Appendices summarize the report's recommendations and offer examples of agency innovations and resources for immediate application to improving performance management in agencies throughout the government.

Theme 1: Expect Excellence

Communicate Expectations
- Employees need a clear picture of what is expected of them, both as individuals and as members of a team, if appropriate.
- Communicating clear expectations is an ongoing responsibility for senior management as well as supervisors and team leaders.
- Employees should understand how their contributions—and their colleagues' contributions—link to the organization's mission and program goals.

- Performance plans for Senior Executive Service and General Schedule employees should correlate directly to the agency's Annual Performance Plan and other departmental and component strategic and operating plans.
- Agencies should monitor performance to ensure that progress is being made and expectations will be met, making mid-course corrections as things change. For example, under the Social Security Administration's two-level performance assessment program, employees have noted that mandatory informal discussions between managers and employees are the best part of the process.
- Agencies that use balanced measures of results—operations results, customer satisfaction, and employees' perceptions of their workplace—are achieving real breakthroughs in how they plan and communicate expectations.
- Shared performance expectations, established jointly through supervisors and employees and management and unions working in partnership, lead to greater understanding and ownership of the work to be done and improve the chances for success.

What employees tell us: In the 1999 NPR Employee Survey, only one out of four respondents reported that they had a clear understanding of how "good performance" is defined in their agency.

Recommendations

- Agencies should update their employee performance plans, using balanced measures extensively and working with their labor partners in a constructive discussion about effective, credible measurement.
- Employee plans should be linked to the goals of their respective offices (e.g., as expressed in agency strategic plans and the Annual Performance Plan under the Government Performance and Results Act).
- Agencies should emphasize monitoring performance and giving employees ongoing, timely, and honest feedback (beyond a required progress review) to help sustain and reinforce what is expected.
- The Administration should pursue changes to the performance management statute that will emphasize improving performance and results through setting goals and objectives for organizational, group, and individual performance, as well as increasing flexibility for agencies to provide rewards to employees to recognize and encourage improved performance and results.

Create a Climate for Excellence

- Federal leaders and managers create a climate for excellence by communicating their vision, values, and expectations clearly.
- Expecting excellence sets the direction.
- But getting there and staying there requires a climate—led from the top—that sustains excellence.
- In an organization with a climate for excellence, high standards and continuous improvement become the "norm."
- Those high standards keep everyone's gaze upward toward the horizon and away from a bureaucratic minimum.

- By emphasizing excellence and improvement, performance management's focus shifts away from simply labeling employees in a meaningless ritual.
- Management plays an important role by recognizing excellence— quickly and repeatedly—because recognition affects two sets of employees:
  - The employees who receive the recognition, and
  - The employees who observe the recognition and learn what is valued.

What employees tell us: In the 1999 NPR Employee Survey, only two out of five respondents were satisfied with the recognition they receive for doing a good job.

Recommendations

- Senior management should provide visible support to their agency's performance culture and climate for excellence (e.g., with a top-level "performance counts" statement, as well as day-to-day support).
- Agencies must establish and communicate clear goals and develop effective performance measures that are consistent and balanced.
- Agencies should make sure that the resources (technology, learning, information) employees and their leaders need to do an excellent job are available.
- Formal and informal recognition programs should be linked to desired performance outcomes.
- Agencies should recognize that individuals differ in reaction to performance management techniques and should permit supervisors flexibility in meeting individual needs.
- Agencies should be committed to developing the tools and competencies (i.e., knowledge, skills, abilities, and attributes) that will let employees excel; for example, by offering comprehensive training and continuing professional development in essential employee and leadership skills, as well as by maintaining a library of readily accessible employee development tools.
- Agencies should consider establishing comprehensive leadership development programs that assure a continuous supply of highly qualified managers.
- Agencies should be committed to helping each other by sharing their formal and informal performance management practices and experiences through a clearinghouse at the Performance Management Technical Assistance Center on the OPM Web site.

Theme 2: Establish Accountability

Hold Supervisors Accountable for Managing Performance

- Employees are accountable for being results-oriented and customer-focused; in turn, they hold their leaders, managers, and colleagues accountable for achieving excellence.
- Supervisors and team leaders must see performance management as a central role, not a collateral duty.
- By "walking the talk," executives can model effective performance management for managers and supervisors, for example, by starting with an overall assessment of organizational performance.
- Supervisors' and team leaders' "excellence" in performance management needs to be expected, developed, assessed, and recognized at least as much as their technical excellence.
- Using balanced measures offers an opportunity to provide employee feedback about how well their performance is managed.

- Managers should commend supervisors and team leaders for managing performance well.

What employees tell us: In the 1999 NPR Employee Survey, only half of the respondents reported that their immediate supervisor or team leader was doing a good or very good job.

Recommendations

- Agencies should share their successful practices and resources that keep supervisors managing performance effectively.
- Agencies should emphasize training in basic performance management skills; for example, by conducting intensive training for all new managers, supervisors, and team leaders on giving performance feedback and ensuring that all leaders receive updated training on performance feedback at least bi-annually.
- Agencies should make managing performance effectively a central factor in evaluating managerial and supervisory performance.

Include Performance Management Outcomes in HR Accountability Systems

- The Government's Merit Systems Principles include the following performance management principles that each agency is accountable for using its human resources management systems to support:
  - Excellence in performance should be rewarded.
  - Employees whose performance does not improve to meet established standards should be separated.
- The HR accountability systems that agencies are developing under the leadership of the Office of Personnel Management should examine how well the agency is achieving outcomes such as:
  - Positive linkages between performance and rewards, especially financial incentives;
  - Positive improvements in systems that proactively prevent performance deficiencies from developing in the first place; and
  - Customer and employee perceptions that poor performance is addressed and dealt with effectively.

Recommendations

- Agencies should establish tracking systems for performance management data and interventions and use this information to improve the effectiveness of their performance management programs.
- Agencies should examine how effectively performance management practices are integrated and aligned in support of mission accomplishment by examining and correlating agency information on Annual Performance Plan results, SES performance bonuses, performance ratings of record, and budget.
- Agencies should evaluate the effectiveness of their awards programs and, as appropriate, re-engineer them to focus on rewarding and publicizing tangible accomplishments at the individual or organizational level that improve products or customer service or otherwise directly contribute to achieving strategic goals and objectives.

- Agencies should share their success stories at reinvigorating their performance management programs and practices, both formal and informal.

Theme 3: Take Timely Action

Intervene Early
- Experience, particularly at the executive levels, indicates that resolving a "performance problem" may be a matter of creating a better fit between the employee and the role she or he is expected to perform.
  - Some employees who fail to perform well may be underutilized, and
  - Some may be performing functions that grew out of job restructuring, reassignments, downsizing or automation that the employees are not prepared to perform due to lack of training, skills, etc.
- The old adage that "an ounce of prevention is worth a pound of cure" applies particularly well to anticipating the productivity impact of introducing new technologies and to dealing with performance problems.
  - When significant new responsibilities or technological skills are added, training that precedes implementation can help keep performance from slipping.
  - It takes far fewer resources to identify and correct performance that is starting to slip, than to intervene after a downward spiral has continued over months or even years.
  - Employees are often relieved and much more responsive to counseling and support when it is offered early.
- Timely and concerted action gets the best results.
  - Putting together a set of resources (e.g., from the training, employee relations, and employee assistance programs, as well as other staff offices and the line organization) can help the supervisor identify, accurately diagnose, and address a performance problem quickly.

What employees tell us: In the 1999 NPR Employee Survey, only 28 percent of respondents reported that corrective actions were taken with poor performers.

Recommendations

- Agencies should share successful techniques for designing and supplying proactive performance support, particularly in situations where new technologies and job duties are being introduced.
- Agencies should share successful early intervention practices.
- Agencies should make the modest investment to provide supervisors with more tools for at-the-desk, just-in-time help, such as the interactive CD-ROM on resolving performance problems that is available from the Office of Personnel Management.
- Agencies should work with unions to develop simplified, effective, and fair alternative dispute resolution (ADR) alternatives to the current statutory process for dealing with poor performers.
- Agencies should share their resources, especially specific training for managers to use ADR techniques and to overcome their natural resistance to confrontation.

Support Supervisors Taking Performance-Based Actions

- Because performance problems are relatively uncommon, most supervisors are not "practiced hands" at dealing with the full set of procedures and require support from several perspectives:
  - Many supervisors are convinced that they should be acting on the problem, but are equally convinced that senior management will fail to support them.
  - A performance-based action is a legal process that has specific requirements.
  - Many supervisors have concerns about their personal liability.
  - Most supervisors need some moral and emotional support to get through what will never be a pleasant part of their job.
- Top management should commit the necessary resources and support; any failure to do so will have a chilling effect on the agency's managers and supervisors.
- The Human Resources Office must be ready and able to help; in some instances this may require getting support from other agencies.
- Some agencies have streamlined their own internally imposed agency processes.
- Every effort should be made to improve the government wide process for taking performance-based actions where possible, while maintaining employee protections.

What managers tell us: In the 1999 SES Survey, nearly one out of three respondents cited lack of upper management support as the reason they had not terminated a poor performer.

Recommendations

- The Administration should pursue changes to the performance management laws that will simplify the process for removing poor performers while preserving due process protections.
- Agencies should share successful practices for giving managers and supervisors the support that leads to successful resolutions.
- Agencies should pilot multi-party (i.e., "SWAT" or "Rapid Response" team) approaches to dealing with poor performers.

This report carries a simple message about performance management—in the federal government, leaders, managers, and employees have a mutual obligation to provide value and excellence to America.

The answers are within our grasp:

- Review and re-review your expectations so both manager and employee will clearly understand what it takes to deliver that value and excellence.
- Establish a contract with your employee laying out those expectations clearly.
- Develop the necessary performance management skills for coaching, assisting, measuring, recognizing, etc.
- Provide appropriate ongoing feedback and follow-up, both positive and negative.
- Reward the great performers, and move or otherwise deal with the poor performers.

Leadership is the key!

Appendix A—Summary of Recommendations

Theme 1: Expect Excellence

- Agencies should update their employee performance plans, using balanced measures extensively and working with their labor partners in a constructive discussion about effective, credible measurement.
- Employee plans should be linked to the goals of their respective offices (e.g., as expressed in agency strategic plans and the Annual Performance Plan under the Government Performance and Results Act).
- Agencies should emphasize monitoring performance and giving employees ongoing, timely, and honest feedback (beyond a required progress review) to help sustain and reinforce what's expected.
- The Administration should pursue changes to the performance management statute that will emphasize improving performance and results through setting goals and objectives for organizational, group, and individual performance, as well as increasing flexibility for agencies to provide rewards to employees to recognize and encourage improved performance and results.
- Senior management should provide visible support to their agency's performance culture and climate for excellence (e.g., with a top-level "performance counts" statement, as well as day-to-day support).
- Agencies must establish and communicate clear goals and develop effective performance measures that are consistent and balanced.
- Agencies should make sure that the resources (technology, learning, information) employees and their leaders need to do an excellent job are available.
- Formal and informal recognition programs should be linked to desired performance outcomes.
- Agencies should recognize that individuals differ in reaction to performance management techniques and should permit supervisors flexibility in meeting individual needs.
- Agencies should be committed to developing the tools and competencies (i.e., knowledge, skills, abilities, and attributes) that will let employees excel; for example, by offering comprehensive training and continuing professional development in essential employee and leadership skills, as well as by maintaining a library of readily accessible employee development tools.
- Agencies should consider establishing comprehensive leadership development programs that assure a continuous supply of highly qualified managers.
- Agencies should be committed to helping each other by sharing their formal and informal performance management practices and experiences through a clearinghouse at the Performance Management Technical Assistance Center on the OPM Web site.

Theme 2: Establish Accountability

- Agencies should share their successful practices and resources that keep supervisors managing performance effectively.
- Agencies should emphasize training in basic performance management skills; for example, by conducting intensive training for all new managers, supervisors, and team leaders on giving performance feedback and ensuring that all leaders receive updated training on performance feedback at least bi-annually.
- Agencies should make managing performance effectively a central factor in evaluating managerial and supervisory performance.

- Agencies should establish tracking systems for performance management data and interventions and use this information to improve the effectiveness of their performance management programs.
- Agencies should examine how effectively performance management practices are integrated and aligned in support of mission accomplishment by examining and correlating agency information on Annual Performance Plan results, SES performance bonuses, performance ratings of record, and budget.
- Agencies should evaluate the effectiveness of their awards programs and, as appropriate, re-engineer them to focus on rewarding and publicizing tangible accomplishments at the individual or organizational level that improve products or customer service or otherwise directly contribute to achieving strategic goals and objectives.
- Agencies should share their success stories at reinvigorating their performance management programs and practices, both formal and informal.

Theme 3: Take Timely Action

- Agencies should share successful techniques for designing and supplying proactive performance support, particularly in situations where new technologies and job duties are being introduced.
- Agencies should share successful early intervention practices.
- Agencies should make the modest investment to provide supervisors with more tools for at-the-desk, just-in-time help, such as the interactive CD-ROM on resolving performance problems that is available from the Office of Personnel Management.
- Agencies should work with unions to develop simplified, effective, and fair alternative dispute resolution (ADR) alternatives to the current statutory process for dealing with poor performers.
- Agencies should share their resources, especially specific training for managers to use ADR techniques and to overcome their natural resistance to confrontation.
- The Administration should pursue changes to the performance management laws that will simplify the process for removing poor performers while preserving due process protections.
- Agencies should share successful practices for giving managers and supervisors the support that leads to successful resolutions.
- Agencies should pilot multi-party (i.e., "SWAT" or "Rapid Response" team) approaches to dealing with poor performers.

Appendix B—Agency Innovations and Resources

Theme 1: Expect Excellence

Communicate expectations

- At the Department of Education, Senior Officers' performance plans are tied to the strategic goals of the agency and subordinate managers' and supervisors' performance plans are being revised to support those goals.
- The Department of Commerce will soon launch a standardized set of performance measures for SES managers. Each senior executive will have three standard elements consistent across the department in areas such as Leadership and Diversity, and two elements that relate directly to the department's or bureau's Strategic Plans. This will promote

greater linkages with more direct results being realized as well as provide a method to assess and compare executive performance across the department. In addition, the relationship between financial recognition/bonuses will be greatly enhanced.

- In 1998, the Department of Commerce conducted a review of linkages between the department's Strategic Plan, bureau operating plans, and SES performance plans. This review concluded that a more consistent approach, including balanced measures and direct Strategic Plan linkages, was necessary. The result was SES 2000, an innovative program designed to revitalize the SES within the Department of Commerce as well as strengthen the corporate utilization of SES resources. SES 2000 emphasizes increased executive development, improved succession planning and SES candidate development, more robust SES performance management policies and practices, and greater communications with the SES corps.
- Before completing SES performance reviews, senior officials at the Department of Commerce convey to bureau leadership how well the bureau, overall, has performed for the previous year. This information is then factored into SES performance evaluations.
- The National Treasury Employees Union and the Office of the Secretary and Administration on Aging (Department of Health and Human Services) have just signed a memorandum of understanding for a pilot of a two-tier performance evaluation program. Recognizing how critical feedback skills are for successful performance management, the agreement calls for training both supervisors AND employees in how to give and request constructive feedback.
- At the Department of Transportation, a Balanced Scorecard is used for measuring performance in many of the support offices including acquisition and procurement, human resources, and real and property management.
- The Department of Transportation has adopted seven recommendations from an Accountability Workgroup to improve individual accountability throughout the department including cascading the performance agreements to all SES members in the department. The department has a performance management framework that links employee performance at all levels to the DOT strategic plan.
- The Department of Transportation uses Performance Agreements linked to the goals in the DOT Performance Plan between the Secretary and senior officials and has regular monthly meetings between the Deputy Secretary and Administrators to track progress against the goals in the agreements.
- At the Social Security Administration, senior executives' and higher level management officials' performance plans are linked to key SSA initiatives which are related to GPRA. Lower level employees' performance plans are linked to the goals of their respective offices.
- The Department of the Interior has established a Performance Management Council to guide the development of Interior's strategic planning process. This group is composed of senior planning officials from each bureau, as well as representatives from the departmental management offices.
- The Bureau of Land Management (Department of the Interior) has redesigned its budget development and execution process to be the main communication tool with employees and managers of the organizational expectations. By providing budget targets 1 year in advance, the field units are able to negotiate their level of performance based on the available human and fiscal resources and realign, if necessary, their priorities and skill mix to meet the organizational needs.
- At the Bureau of Land Management (Department of the Interior), Senior Executive Service personnel performance evaluations are based on the agency's strategic goal areas, and lower-level managers' evaluations are based on the SES criteria.

- At the Department of the Interior, Superintendents of the National Park Service are evaluated, in part, on their performance against their park-specific GPRA annual performance plan.
- At the Department of the Interior, the development of employee performance plans has been streamlined. One goal was to restrict the construction of detailed written performance standards to the small percentage of employees who are having performance problems. [Note: OPM's legislative proposals are specifically designed to facilitate this approach.]
- Performance contracts or performance agreements are negotiated between the manager and the employee at NASA.
- NASA also uses an automated assessment tool that links an individual's performance plan and accomplishments to the strategic plan and GPRA.
- Performance management seminars (3-day courses) are held at the Department of State's Foreign Service Institute four times a year. Participants learn to write and communicate clear performance plans, provide coaching and feedback to improve performance, and conduct effective performance appraisals.
- The NPR Report on *Balancing Measures: Best Practices in Performance Management*, available on the NPR Web site, offers practical advice about how to develop and implement balanced measures of results. In addition, it provides extensive examples and contacts from the public and private sector.
- A series of articles on *Improved Performance Starts with Planning*, originally published in OPM's bi-monthly newsletter *Workforce Performance*, are available at the Performance Management Technical Assistance Center on the OPM Web site.
- OPM's *Measuring Employee Performance: Aligning Employee Performance Plans with Organizational Goals* workshop/handbook covers an eight-step process for developing employee performance plans that are aligned with and support organizational goals from Results Act Strategic and Annual Performance Plans. The Handbook, which is available at the Performance Management Technical Assistance Center on the OPM Web site, provides guidelines for writing performance elements and standards along with hands-on exercises to give users a chance to practice their new skills. Agencies such as the U.S. Mint and the National Institute for Standards and Technology ensure that all their managers are trained in this method.
- Checklists for good performance plans are available on the OPM Web site.

Create a climate for excellence
- At the Treasury Department, agency leadership identifies priority areas and communicates them to the department's bureaus for action.
- The Department of Transportation provides Partnering for Excellence training.
- The Department of Transportation flagship initiative for Learning and Development encourages increased training opportunities and incentives, including a budgeted employee training pool for 2001 equaling 2 percent of employee salaries.
- The Department of Transportation has created "Team Excell," an employee team committed to encouraging excellence throughout the department using the Baldrige/Presidential Quality Award criteria as a foundation.
- In 1999, the Department of Education began a program of 40 hours of core curriculum training each year for supervisors, managers, and executives in core competencies and management issues of importance to the department and its principal offices. In addition, all new managers are provided training on the basics of supervision and provided extensive resource materials.
- Based on employee surveys, the Bureau of Land Management (Department of the Interior) has established a series of leadership management and employee development

courses, including a year-long Leadership Academy. The "Leadership Excellence" spectrum of employee, management and leadership training is designed to provide complete and comprehensive training centered around the 27 Senior Executive competencies established by OPM.

- The Bureau of Land Management (Department of the Interior) has established a workforce-planning framework identifying critical skill needs and providing maximum workforce flexibility. The framework calls for each state to analyze its current and future workforce needs and develop a strategy—including alternative delivery mechanisms, such as contracting, term appointments, and sharing scarce skills between different agencies—to address work demands without increasing current permanent staff.

- The "Service First" collaborative partnership between the Bureau of Land Management (Department of the Interior) and the Forest Service (Department of Agriculture) formalizes the agencies' ability to share scarce skills and leverage constrained operations dollars to meet the public's needs and expectations. In the HRM Concept of Operations (www.fs.fed.us/servicefirst), the BLM and the Forest Service have laid out the operational procedures of how the two agencies in two different departments will share employees, accept classifications, and jointly advertise positions.

- Numerous examples of agency practices and programs for successful formal and informal incentive and recognition programs and other effective performance management practices are described in OPM's bi-monthly newsletter *Workforce Performance*. An extensive archive of current and back issues and articles from this newsletter is available at the Performance Management Technical Assistance Center on the OPM Web site.

- *"Label-less" Performance Management Program*—In an effort to dispense with performance "labels" such as "Outstanding" and "Marginal" which tend to attach themselves to employees themselves rather than their performance, the Department of Energy Headquarters now uses a performance evaluation program that summarizes employees' performance as a numerical value. The value is derived by the rating officials comparing an employee's performance of tasks identified for each element (streamlined into very simple "action" statements) against four generic "levels of accomplishment." The elements are weighted according to their critical or non-critical status. The employee's score in each element is multiplied by the assigned level of accomplishment; resulting scores are added and then divided by the weighted number of elements. The resulting value is the employee's rating of record. Both management and the union, the National Treasury Employees Union, have found the new program allows for equitable calculation of performance awards and allows the employees to see the direct effects of their performance on individual elements.

- *Multiple Progress Reviews Requirements*—Department of Energy Headquarters and its bargaining unit representative, the National Treasury Employees Union (NTEU), are not only encouraging employees and managers to discuss employees' day-to-day tasks and requirements, but also the employees' role in the success of the larger organization. This will necessarily require more communications—more instruction and feedback—than under the previous program. Accordingly, the headquarters performance management program now requires that employee expectations be clarified at the beginning of the performance period, and there must be at least two progress reviews during the period. Progress reviews must be more structured. At each progress review, the rating official must now discuss how the employee's "tasks" (each element has a list of associated tasks) have been performed over the past few months, what documentation supports that performance, and what resources the employee will need in the coming months to support and enhance the employee's and the organization's performance. At the end of each progress review, the employee will be given a non-binding feedback score on each element performed during the progress review period.

Theme 2: Establish Accountability

Hold supervisors accountable for managing performance

- NASA conducts small team reviews of performance plans and assessments to ensure that management responsibilities are addressed.
- The Department of Education has an automated 360-degree performance evaluation system that includes all employees and supervisors, including members of the Senior Executive Service.
- The Indian Health Service (Department of Health and Human Services), as a way to strengthen supervisory skills, is retraining all current supervisors (as well as new ones) in the core interpersonal skills so necessary for good supervision. One large component of the Indian Health Service has gone even further to offer interpersonal skills training to the rest of their employees as well.
- In 2000, the Bureau of Land Management (Department of the Interior) will have all SES and manager appraisals based on its strategic goals and supplemented by a "360-degree review" for developmental purposes.
- The Social Security Administration is planning a competency self-assessment that will include those skills and attributes associated with effective performance management.
- *360-Degree (Upward) Feedback*—Several agencies are using multi-rater assessment techniques to bring their managers, supervisors, and team leaders richer information about their performance. In some cases, the information is used for developmental, rather than evaluative, purposes.
- *The Organizational Assessment Survey*, available through OPM's Personnel Resources and Development Center, measures organizational climate and effectiveness, including the kinds of performance management support that managers provide.

Include performance management outcomes in HR accountability systems

- Performance management has been incorporated into NASA's self-assessment program.
- The Department of the Interior's new human resources accountability system uses a suite of indicators from a wide variety of sources to monitor program performance in the areas covered by the Department's HR Strategic Plan. The system is simple and inexpensive, but effective in producing real-time measures of progress. The system includes performance management outcomes and utilizes a "balanced measures approach."
- OPM's HRM Accountability System Development Guide, which covers the performance management–related Merit System Principles is available on the OPM Web site.
- OPM maintains a clearinghouse of successful and promising applications of HRM accountability systems or their components within federal agencies and other organizations; it is available through OPM's Web site.

Theme 3: Take Timely Action

Intervene early

- *"Rapid Response Teams"*—The Treasury Department has a Rapid Response Team consisting of several high level staff from the department's personnel and legal headquarters offices. They may be contacted directly by bureau officials to discuss sensitive personnel matters. The team member contacted can work individually, or with another team member, calling on whatever resources are necessary to provide immediate advice and guidance, including options for handling the matter at issue.

- The Department of Health and Human Services reports having success using an informal, multi-party approach to address what they call "underutilization."
- The Department of Education has instituted a mobility assignment program that opens up detail opportunities on a competitive basis (for up to 1 year) to employees throughout the agency. Employees can develop new skills and gain experience that may help qualify them for new positions.
- The Department of Education provides mediation services through its Informal Dispute Resolution Center.
- In 2000, the Department of Education will launch an automated Individual Development Plan system.
- The Department of Transportation secretarial award "Find the Good and Praise It" recognizes employee contributions in support of DOT goals. The award is given on a monthly basis.
- NASA uses mandated coaching sessions.
- The Department of the Interior is implementing an early intervention alternative dispute resolution procedure called CORE, which is designed to enable a well-trained dispute resolution specialist to intervene in a dispute at an early stage to assist the parties in resolving the current misunderstanding and to help them develop conflict resolution skills to facilitate their future dealings. While this process will be open to any dispute an employee brings forward, experience suggests that a great many of these disputes involve performance expectations and performance appraisal issues.
- *Performance Development Resources (PDR)*—A Navy demonstration project includes a process in which a pool of people, including union representatives, act as a support system for employees and managers throughout the performance process. Should performance problems arise, PDR can be particularly useful in diagnosing issues impacting performance and identifying options for addressing these issues, for example, development opportunities, tools to support improved performance, and reassignment of the employee to a position that better matches his/her capabilities and interests. PDR may also identify systemic or organization wide issues that may be affecting performance. Supervisors are expected to use PDR for assistance in preventing and alleviating performance problems. Employees may also use PDR to assist them in correcting self-identified performance problems, in development planning, and to facilitate communication and feedback with their supervisors. [Note: Although PDR is part of a demonstration project, it can be implemented without obtaining waivers of law or regulation.]
- The Social Security Administration has invested in training for managers to *overcome resistance to confrontation.*
- Training in subjects like performance counseling and dealing with difficult people is available from a variety of private vendors.
- Several agencies use a checklist for successful interventions.
- The comprehensive *Alternative Dispute Resolution (ADR) Resource Guide* is available on OPM's Web site. ADR consists of a variety of approaches to early intervention and dispute resolution. Many of these approaches include the use of a neutral individual such as a mediator who can assist disputing parties in resolving their disagreements. ADR increases the parties' opportunities to resolve disputes prior to or during the use of formal administrative procedures and litigation (which can be very costly and time-consuming). The Guide provides an overall picture of how the most common forms of ADR are being implemented in federal agencies. It summarizes a number of current ADR programs (including alternative discipline programs), and it includes descriptions of shared neutrals programs where agencies have collaborated to reduce the costs of ADR.

It provides a listing of training and resources available from federal and non-federal sources. It also provides selected ADR-related Web sites. The information in the Guide will be helpful in exploring the feasibility and appropriateness of implementing alternative dispute resolution programs in an organization or enhancing existing programs.

Support supervisors taking performance-based actions

- The various multi-party approaches described above provide continuous support in the event that a performance-based action is pursued.
- "Just in time" training is available for supervisors in the form of OPM's interactive CD-ROM and handbook on *Addressing and Resolving Poor Performance*, which provides direct assistance and advice to supervisors for every stage of the process.
- The Department of Education uses a system of mentoring to provide managers tools and follow-up, as well as a system of executive coaches to work with managers on performance issues.
- At NASA, an agency expert provides performance seminars to field Centers; human resources staff and managers attend.
- The Department of Transportation has a new "Shared Neutrals Program" for timely resolution of conflicts throughout DOT.
- The Department of Commerce prepared, issued, and has posted on its Web site *The Manager's Handbook on Human Resources*. Three chapters in the Handbook pertain to this topic: "How Do I Evaluate an Employee's Performance?" "How Do I Reward an Employee?" and "How Do I Deal with an Employee's Unacceptable Performance." Each chapter provides typical scenarios, principles, where to start, rules and flexibilities, basic steps, needed forms, time frames, good management practices, checklists, and a note on how the SES is different from the GS. The handbook is available at http://ohrm.doc.gov/information/handbook/Mgrhbk.htm.
- The Department of State produced a handbook "Supervisor's Guide—Dealing with Employee Unacceptable Performance and Conduct."
- The Department of State held workshops for all supervisors and managers on how to address unacceptable performance.
- Distance learning approaches can be used to provide management and skills training to address poor performance.
- Sample proposal and decision letters used in pursuing performance actions are available on OPM's Web site.

These additional web sites contain related material on the following topics:

- 1999 NPR Employees Survey (http://www.npr.gov)
- Merit Systems Oversight and Effectiveness Study (http://www.opm.gov/studies/index.htm)
- Performance Management and Incentive Awards (http://www.opm.gov/perform/index.htm)
- Resolving Poor Performance (http://www.opm.gov/perform/poor/index.html-ssi)
- Alternative Dispute Resolution Labor-Management Relations (http://www.opm.gov/er/adrguide/adrhome.html-ssi)
- Labor-Management Relations (http://www.opm.gov/cplmr/index.htm)
- Performance Appraisal in the Senior Executive Service (http://www.opm.gov/ses/appraise.html)
- Management Development Centers (http://www.opm.gov/leader/index.html)

Other items of interest are the Transmittal Memo (http://www.opm.gov/perform/articles/2000/pmcmemo.htm).

CHAPTER 9
Best Practices in Performance Measurement

This chapter presents an excerpt from an article detailing an in-depth study of the use of Balanced Measures in the federal government. It is adapted from the National Partnership for Reinventing Government, "Balancing Measures: Best Practices in Performance Management" (September 1, 1999), www.npr.gov.

BALANCING MEASURES: BEST PRACTICES IN PERFORMANCE MANAGEMENT

Executive Summary

When the Government Performance and Results Act was first implemented, many felt that government management was somehow "different," that the same rules that applied to the private sector could not apply to the public, or at least not in the same way. After all, government agencies do not have a bottom line or profit margin. However, recent efforts, as this study shows repeatedly, attest that is not true. The bottom line for most government organizations is their mission: what they want to achieve.

However, they cannot achieve this mission by managing in a vacuum, any more than can the private sector. More specifically, the roles of customer, stakeholder, and employee in an organization's day-to-day operations are vital to its success—and must be incorporated into that success.

In their groundbreaking *Harvard Business Review* article, Robert S. Kaplan and David P. Norton introduced the concept of the Balanced Scorecard to the private sector. This article, and subsequent works by them, discusses private sector efforts to align corporate initiatives with the need to meet customer and shareholder expectations. This study looks at how these efforts relate to, and are being replicated within, the public sector. It examines the ways and means by which government organizations are trying to include customers, stakeholders, and employees in their performance management efforts—to reach some *balance* among the needs and opinions of these groups along with the achievement of the organization's stated mission. All of the organizations that served as partners in preparing this report have had some level of success in doing this.

Our partners believe that, while there is no perfect fit of the Balanced Scorecard as envisioned by Kaplan and Norton with performance planning, management, and measurement within the public sector, this does not mean that the concept isn't useful in government planning—particularly with some tinkering and tailoring. So, public sector organizations with the most mature strategic planning processes—notably city and state governments—felt that the area of employee satisfaction, for example, translated better to the public sector when seen as employee empowerment and/or involvement.

Defining whom exactly the *customer* is can be a challenge for government agencies, especially for federal agencies with more than one mission. For example, the U.S. Coast Guard has both enforcement and a service mission—and consequently different customer bases. And even those agencies that have but a single mission, such as regulatory agencies like the Environmental Protection Agency, must take into account not only those with whom they deal on a day-to-day basis in their enforcement activities, such as major manufacturers, but also the citizen who is being protected by those enforcement activities. And the organization that provides a service or benefit, like the Social Security Administration, must distinguish between what the customer may want and what U.S. citizens may be willing to spend; that is, to balance their fiscal responsibilities to the taxpayer with their responsibilities to beneficiaries.

Other important lessons about balanced performance measurement gleaned from site visits and interviews with our best practice and resource partners include the following:

- Adapt, do not adopt: Make a best practice work for you.
- We are not so different after all: Public or private, federal, state, or local, there are common problems—and common answers.
- Leadership does not stop at the top, but should cascade throughout an organization, creating champions and a team approach to achievement of mission.
- Listen to your customers and stakeholders.
- Listen to your employees and unions.
- Partnership among customers, stakeholders, and employees results in success. Telling—rather than asking—these groups what they need does not work.

Why should you, a government leader, try to achieve a balanced set of performance measures—or what is often referred to as a *family of measures*? Here's what we found in our research: Because you need to know what your customer's expectations are and what your employee needs to have to meet those expectations. Because you cannot achieve your stated objectives without taking those expectations and needs into account. Most importantly, because it *works*, as can be seen from the success of our partners.

Therefore, you need to balance your mission with customer, stakeholder, and employee perspectives. How exactly do you go about doing this? These are the best practices we learned from our partners.

Establish a Results-Oriented Set of Measures That Balance[s] Business, Customer, and Employee

- *Define what measures mean the most* to customer, stakeholder, and employee by (1) having them work together, (2) creating an easily recognized body of measures, and (3) clearly identifying measures to address their concerns.
- *Commit to initial change* by (1) using expertise wherever you find it; (2) involving everyone in the process; (3) making the system nonpunitive; (4) bringing in the unions; and (5) providing clear, concise guidance as to the establishment, monitoring, and reporting of measures.
- *Maintain flexibility* by (1) recognizing that performance management is a living process, (2) limiting the number of performance measures, and (3) maintaining a balance between financial and nonfinancial measures.

Establish Accountability at All Levels of the Organization

- Lead by example.
- Cascade accountability: share it with the employee by (1) creating a performance-based organization, (2) encouraging sponsorship of measures at all levels, and (3) involving the unions at all levels of performance management.
- Keep the employee informed via intranet and/or Internet; don't rule out alternative forms of communication.
- Keep the customer informed via both the Internet and traditional paper reports.
- Make accountability work: reward employees for success. Supplement or replace monetary rewards with nonmonetary means, reallocate discretionary funds, and base rewards in a team approach.

Collect, Use, and Analyze Data

- *Collect feedback data,* which can be obtained from customers by providing easy access to your organization; remember too that "survey" is not a four-letter word.
- *Collect performance data* by (1) investing both the time and the money to make it right, (2) making sure that your performance data mean something to those that use them, (3) recognizing that everything is not on-line or in one place, and (4) centralizing the data collection function at the highest possible level.
- *Analyze data*: (1) combine feedback and performance data for a more complete picture, (2) conduct root-cause analyses, and (3) make sure everyone sees the results of analyses.

Connect the Dots

If your performance management efforts are not connected to your business plan (which defines day-to-day operations in a government agency) and to the budget (which is where the money is), then you will be doomed to failure because your performance measurement approach will have no real meaning to the people running, or affected by, the program. Planning documents must connect to business plans, and data systems and the budget process must be integrated with all these other factors. By doing so, you can create a strategic management framework which serves to focus the entire organization on the same mission and goals.

Share the Leadership Role

Leadership is a critical element marking successful organizations, both public and private. Cascaded throughout an organization, leadership gives the performance management process a depth and sustainability that survives changes at the top—even those driven by elections and changes in political party leadership. Two experts in the field, the Hon. Maurice McTigue, a former New Zealand cabinet member now working at George Mason University, and Dr. Patricia Ingraham of the Maxwell School at Syracuse University, emphasize in their teaching the importance of leadership in a political environment. Given the potential constraints such an environment can present, a successful public sector organization needs strong leadership that supports the adoption of balanced measures as a feature of organizational management and accountability.

Why Did We Do This Study?

For many years, leaders at all levels in the private and public sectors have searched for the right tools and techniques to help them create high-performing organizations. The Balanced Scorecard introduced in 1992 by Kaplan and Norton of the Harvard Business School galvanized and revolutionized the field. The Balanced Scorecard approach to performance management gained wide use and acclaim in the private sector as a way to build customer and employee data into measuring and ensuring better performance outcomes. It thus transformed the way private sector companies could achieve and analyze high levels of performance and was critical in revitalizing such companies as Federal Express, Corning, and Sears.

In August 1993, Congress passed the Government Performance and Results Act (referred to as both GPRA and the Results Act). Under GPRA, leadership in the public sector was legally obligated to address issues such as performance planning and management—as well as report on the results of those efforts. Many felt that government management was "different," that the rules of performance management and measurement that applied to the private sector could not apply to the public. After all, government agencies do not have a bottom line or profit margin.

Recent efforts have shown, however, that not only do the basic concepts apply to the public sector, they can also be used to create a successful organization. For example, agencies may not have a financial bottom line, but they do have goals and outcomes that can indicate success (e.g., reduction in pollution).

Other concepts apply as well, as was borne out by Executive Order 12862, signed by President Clinton in September 1993. This order requires federal agencies to determine from their customers the kind and quality of service they seek. In the same way that the private sector experienced noticeable changes by measuring beyond business results, government agencies have also begun to balance a greater constellation of measures by incorporating customer needs and expectations into their strategic planning processes. *This balanced approach to performance planning, measurement, and management is helping government agencies achieve results Americans—whether customers, stakeholders, employees, or other—actually care about.*

Cities, states, and counties have actively adapted the balanced measures approach. Some federal organizations too have begun to pursue balanced measurement as part of ongoing efforts to improve efficiency, effectiveness, and customer service in their organizations. Abroad, similar activities have been taking place. The British government formed the Performance and Innovation Unit to, among other things, "promote innovative solutions that improved the effectiveness of policy, the quality of services and the responsiveness to users' needs." Also, the Service First Unit in the UK has been focusing on customer service issues for several years. Many Canadian government agencies—including Natural Resources Canada, the St. Lawrence Seaway Management Corporation, Atomic Energy of Canada, Ltd., and the Trademarks Office—have been working to link their customer service, performance management, and budget processes together.

At a time when new performance, budget, and strategic challenges to the public sector affect its current and future decisions, much can be gleaned from these various experiences with balanced performance measurement. Thus, Vice President Al Gore—after hearing three highly successful and diverse corporate leaders at a reinvention forum attribute balanced measurement of performance as critical to taking their companies to the top—charged the National Partnership for Reinventing Government (NPR) with identifying and studying best practices in using balanced measures in the public and private sectors.

Lessons We Learned

Overall, a balanced approach to performance measurement works and will improve organizational performance when used. Flexibility is the key. There is no "cookie cutter" approach, but there are elements and experiences reported here that can be useful and beneficial to all agencies.

- *Adapt, don't adopt.* A best practice generally cannot be adopted exactly the way it was done in another organization, but it can be adapted to fit your organizational needs and culture. Most of the organizations we interviewed have adapted the traditional Balanced Scorecard into a family of measures that is uniquely suited to their culture, their structure, their mission. In the final analysis, you must adapt an approach to fit *your* particular needs.
- *We aren't so different after all.* One of the most interesting discoveries for the team was the fact that the problems the different organizations were facing were not very different. Most struggled with the same issues: reducing the number of measures, validating and verifying data, establishing accountability and responsibility without being punitive, and—most importantly—trying to balance achievement of the organization's mission with the needs of customer, stakeholder, and employee. In many cases, merely defining the customer was an obstacle. Public or private, federal, state, or local, there are common problems—and common answers—in many areas.
- *Leadership doesn't stop at the top.* Leadership is important, but not just at the top levels; leadership by employees in solving problems and achieving mission is what makes for a most successful organization.
- *Listen to your customers and stakeholders.* You might be surprised to learn what is really important to them. The Oregon Department of Motor Vehicles was prepared to spend money on ways to provide faster service and shorter lines. Then it asked its customers what they wanted. *They* wanted a choice in the ID picture that would be laminated onto their license. Oregon listened and invested in better photographic equipment and provided a choice to the customer as to the picture to be used.
- *Listen to your employees and unions.* Employees have historical knowledge and experience at the day-to-day operations level. Don't underestimate the importance of this information and expertise. In addition, regarding the union, if it is part of the solution, it is no longer part of the problem. This precept is especially critical in achieving culture change within an organization.
- *Partner with customers, stakeholders and employees; don't control.* The more you partner with those who have a vested interest in the success of your organization, the more successful your organization is likely to be. Some of the most successful organizations work closely not only with customers and employees, but also with unions and legislators. Better communication results in an increased level of trust.

Most importantly, we learned that *there is no such thing as a fixed and truly balanced set of measures*; instead, the *process* of balancing the needs of customers and employees against mission is a constant and living one, flexible and open to change.

The team learned a great deal from this study; we are pleased to share this knowledge with you. The practices listed here can be used, adapted, and implemented throughout the public sector. We hope this report will be seen as a tool to help everyone do their job better and more efficiently.

Balancing Measures: Why Should I Do It and What Does It Mean?

> Reflecting back on the long history of federal service, I never saw any single measure which could adequately describe an agency's performance. Use of the "scorecard," because it balances both internal and external stakeholder concerns, gives us a much more comprehensive, and balanced, picture of how we are doing. The measures we traditionally used tended to focus almost exclusively on internal processes. They also failed to measure three major areas: the real cost of doing business, the impact of the processes on the veteran-customer, and their impact on employees. Use of the scorecard balances our measures because it looks at both external and internal measures. They keep the organization focused on the vision and our stakeholders: veteran-customers, employees, and tax-payers. The scorecard measures provide a "line of sight" for every employee to see their contribution to organizational results.
> —Joe Thompson, Under Secretary for Benefits,
> Veterans Benefits Administration, Department of Veterans Affairs

Balancing measures is a strategic management system for achieving long-term goals. Senior executives in industries from banking and oil to insurance and retailing use balanced measures to guide current performance and plan future performance. They use measures in four categories—financial performance, customer knowledge, internal business processes, and learning and growth—to align individual, organizational, and cross-departmental initiatives and to identify processes for meeting customer and shareholder objectives.

Their experience has shown that *balancing a family of performance measures works*. This means that in each phase of performance planning, management, and measurement, the customer, stakeholder, and employee are considered in balance with the need to achieve a specific mission or result. This approach has worked in the private sector and is beginning to take firm root in government as well. While there is no exact formula for applying balanced measures, the goal of this report is to provide options and courses of action for use in and across the federal government. The experiences of those who have begun to use balanced measures provide opportunities for agencies to read about what has been successful for others, to choose applicable practices, and to improve performance to match the best in the business.

Are You a Driver or a Pilot? Instrument Panel versus Dashboard

Using balanced measures allows you to mirror the factors that you believe are critical to the success of your organization. "A good way to understand the balanced scorecard is to imagine yourself as the captain of a jumbo jet," write Robert Kaplan and David Norton in their groundbreaking article on the management tool in the *Harvard Business Review*. They continue:

> Imagine the flight deck and all the instruments, dials and gauges on the panel in front of you. These instruments tell you about the various parts of the plane and how it is flying. Reliance on the altimeter only would be foolish—you might know your altitude, but you would not have any warning about impending storms. You wouldn't look only at the radar, of course—how would you know when you were low on fuel?

Balanced measures serve as an *instrument panel* for your organization. They provide important information from different perspectives, creating a holistic view of the organization's health. They bring together on a single management report many of the disparate elements of the organization's agenda.

Another useful metaphor in discussing a balanced approach to performance management is the ***dashboard approach***. Management, when resistant to change, will often complain that it cannot focus on everything at once, that the "powers that be" need to make up their mind about exactly what it is the leader is to look at. The answer to this is that being a good leader is like driving a car. After all, there are many gauges on the dashboard. While you are driving, you take note of the level of fuel (you don't want to run out of gas). You watch the water level (you wouldn't want to overheat the engine). In addition, if an emergency light were to come on, you would notice that as well. These all are secondary observations, however, to the driver's primary focus of moving the car safely in one direction while watching for obstacles in the road, including other drivers. That is exactly what a good leader in an organization should be doing. A balanced set of performance measures is like the gauges on the car; the mission is the destination.

Why a Balanced Approach?

Regardless of which metaphor you embrace, a balanced approach allows you to consider all the important operational measures at the same time, letting you see whether improvement in one area is achieved at the expense of another. Key indicators should tell you how the organization is doing. They will probably change over time to reflect shifting organizational goals. Performance levels can be reported on a monthly or quarterly basis. All levels of management, including field personnel, can participate in the reporting process; together, they provide a good idea of the health of the organization from a variety of perspectives. It is only with a balanced approach that leaders can create success throughout their organizations.

This proven approach to strategic management imbeds long-term strategy into the management system through the mechanism of measurement. It translates vision and strategy into a tool that effectively communicates strategic intent, and motivates and tracks performance against established goals.

A strategy is a shared understanding about how a goal is to be reached. Balancing measures allows management to translate the strategy into a clear set of objectives. These objectives are then further translated into a system of performance measurements that effectively communicates a powerful, forward-looking, strategic focus to the entire organization. In contrast with traditional, financially based measurement systems, ***the balanced measures approach solidifies an organization's focus on future success by setting objectives and measuring performance from distinct perspectives.*** The old method of management, which focused only on the bottom line, no longer works. If the customer, stakeholder, and employee are not part of the solution, they will forever be part of the problem.

Balanced across What Perspectives?

You need to look at your performance management from three perspectives: employee, customer, and business.

The ***employee perspective*** focuses attention on the performance of the key internal processes that drive the organization. This perspective directs attention to the basis of all future success—the organization's people and infrastructure. Adequate investment in these areas is critical to all long-term success. Without employee buy-in, an organization's achievements will be minimal. Employees must be part of the team.

Examples of Concerns from the Employee Perspective
- How do you get employees to see the federal government as an employer of choice?
- Focus on issues such as employee development and retention.

The *customer perspective* considers the organization's performance through the eyes of a customer, so that the organization retains a careful focus on customer needs and satisfaction. For a government entity, this perspective takes on a somewhat different meaning than for a private sector firm; that is because most public sector organizations have many types of customers. The private sector recognizes the importance of the customer and makes the customer a driver of performance. To achieve the best in business performance, the government, too, must incorporate customer needs, wants, and must respond to them as part of its performance planning.

Examples of Concerns from the Customer Perspective
- How do you want your customers to view you?
- Who are your customers? Is there more than one group?
- Are measures based on external customer input?
- Do your measures reflect the characteristics of good service (accessible, accurate, clear, closure, timely, respectful)?

The *business perspective*, like the customer perspective, has a different interpretation in the government than in the private sector. For many organizations, there are actually two separate sets of measures: the *outcomes*, or social/political impacts, which define the role of the agency/department within the government and American society; and the *business processes* needed for organizational efficiency and effectiveness.

Examples of Business Results
- How do you want your stakeholders and/or customers to view you?
- Are your measures outcome/results-based?
- Are the results something customers care about?
- Do you have real-time data for reporting purposes?

Together, these perspectives provide a balanced view of the present and future performance of the organization. A balanced set of measures allows leaders to think of their organization in its totality. *There is no one "right" family of measures.* The measures must reflect the overall mission strategy of the organization. They have to be the measures that drive the organization. In most cases, they are developed through an iterative, evolutionary process. You can have as many categories as you want, but the idea is to keep it as simple as possible so that your measurements can be global and quick.

For the team members of this study, the key challenge has been to determine what has to happen to make it possible for government leaders to manage through the use of a balanced set of measures.

Summary of Best Practices in Balancing Measures

In 1994, Vice President Al Gore gave a lecture as part of the Georgetown University Series on Governmental Reform in which he identified the characteristics of "The New Job of the

Federal Executive." Among those characteristics were "creating a team environment, empowering employees, putting customers first, and communicating with employees." Those characteristics are embedded in the best practices of our partners—especially in this area of performance measurement.

There is no generic set of balanced measures that can be applied as best practice to all functions of the public sector. Certain conditions, however, need to exist within an organization for a balanced approach to performance management to be successful:

- Strong leadership that supports the adoption of balanced measures as a feature of organizational management and accountability;
- The capability to communicate effectively throughout the organization and the organization's ability to communicate to decision makers; and
- The knowledge that customers, employees, and stakeholders are fully informed and that they understand and support the initiatives of the organization.

While an attempt to find a *one-size-fits-all* approach will not work, there are some generic principles that remain constant across all government organizations:

- *Good product or service.* Does the organization meet the consumer's need for goods or services or rectify a perceived wrong?
- *Good image.* How does public opinion view the organization? Are employees enthused by the public's perception of them?
- *Good availability.* Can customers get easy access and satisfaction? Is the organization ready and able to respond immediately to any reasonable challenge?
- *Good employer.* Are there high levels of staff retention, staff morale, and job satisfaction?
- *Continuous improvement.* Is there a continuous evaluation process to identify and implement improvements? Do the improvements benefit the product to the community?

A successful organization in the public sector will apply these principles to its strategic framework, which links performance planning, measurement, and reporting to day-to-day operations, balancing the need to achieve a stated mission with the needs of the customer, stakeholder, and employee. . . . [O]ur partners are doing just this as they:

- Establish a results-oriented set of measures that balances business, customer, and employee;
- Establish accountability at all levels of the organization;
- Collect, use, and analyze data;
- Connect the dots; and
- Share the leadership role.

CHAPTER 10

The Balanced Scorecard in Information Technology at the General Services Administration

One of the best sources of basic information on the Balanced Scorecard is the General Services Administration (GSA) guide on information technology (IT). The guide was published early in the process of applying the Balanced Scorecard to federal government operations.

There are few, if any, more important areas in the federal government than the effective application of IT. And yet, the area has been plagued with delays and cost overruns over the past several decades. This detailed GSA document is full of good examples of how the Balanced Scorecard can be used to more effectively develop and deploy this technology.

EIGHT STEPS TO DEVELOP AND USE INFORMATION TECHNOLOGY PERFORMANCE MEASURES EFFECTIVELY

The following material was adapted from the Office of Government Wide Policy, General Services Administration, "Eight Steps To Develop and Use Information Technology Performance Measures Effectively," Washington, D.C., GSA, December 1996.

Introduction

The federal government spends over $25 billion annually on IT systems and services. Do these systems and services improve service to the public? Do these systems and services improve productivity or reduce costs of federal agencies? Without measuring and communicating the results, how will anyone know?

For the remainder of this decade and into the next century, the federal government will decrease in size as government balances the federal budget. IT will play a significant role in making the federal government more efficient and effective as it downsizes. The Clinger-Cohen Act requires each executive agency to establish a process to select, manage, and evaluate the results of their IT investments; report annually to Congress on progress made toward agency goals; and link IT performance measures to agency programs.

The Clinger-Cohen Act evolved from a report by Senator Cohen of Maine, entitled "Computer Chaos." In the report, Senator Cohen identified major projects that wasted billions of dollars because of poor management. To improve the success of IT projects in the federal sector, Senator Cohen stated the government needs to do better up-front planning of IT projects particularly when they define objectives, analyze alternatives, and establish performance measures that link to agency accomplishments.

This publication provides an approach to develop and implement IT performance measures in concert with guidance provided by OMB and GAO. It cites and explains an eight-step process to link IT investments to agency accomplishments that meets the requirements of the Clinger-Cohen Act and the Government Performance and Results Act (GPRA).

Congress and OMB emphasize performance measures as a requirement to receive funding. Soon, agency funding levels will be determined to a large degree on the projected results of IT investments and the measures selected to verify the results. This guide presents a systematic approach for developing and using IT performance measures to improve results.

The eight-step approach focuses on up-front planning using the Balanced Scorecard. IT performance measures will be effective if agencies adequately plan and link their IT initiatives to their strategies. The Balanced Scorecard translates strategy into action. The eight-step approach is a logical sequence of tasks. In practice, some steps can be combined. Because performance measurement is an iterative process, agencies should expect to apply the eight steps repeatedly to obtain effective performance measures and improve performance.

Principles of Step 1

- Establish clear linkage, define specific business goals and objectives
- Secure senior management commitment and involvement
- Identify stakeholders and customers and nurture consensus

Step 1: Link Information Technology Projects to Agency Goals and Objectives

The process to effectively measure the contribution of IT projects to mission results begins with a clear understanding of an agency's goals and objectives. Linking IT projects to agency goals and objectives increases the likelihood that results will contribute to agency accomplishments. Accordingly, this linkage improves an agency's ability to measure the contribution of IT projects to mission accomplishments.

Accomplishments are positive results that achieve an organization's goals and objectives. Because information system (IS) organizations and IT projects support the mission and programs, the organization's vision and business strategies need to be established before IT projects can be linked to goals and objectives. To establish clear linkage, strategic plans need to define specific business goals and objectives and incorporate IT as a strategic resource.

The GPRA requires executive agencies to develop strategic plans and performance measures for major programs. Each strategic business unit (SBU) should have a strategic plan. An SBU is an internal organization that has a mission and customers distinct from other segments of the enterprise. Processing disability claim requests, launching satellites, or maintaining military aircraft are examples of SBUs.

As important as strategic plans can be, they often are forgotten soon after prepared because they don't translate well into action. In most cases, business strategies reflect lofty objectives ("Be our customers' number one supplier."), which are nearly impossible to translate into day-to-day activities. Also, strategic plans typically focus 3 to 5 years into the future in contrast with performance measures, which focus on ongoing operations. This difference in focus causes confusion, and sometimes conflict, for line managers and program managers.

The Balanced Scorecard (BSC) is a framework that helps organizations translate business strategies into action. Originally developed for private industry, the BSC balances short- and long-term objectives. Private industry routinely uses financial measures to assess performance although financial measures focus only on the short term, particularly the results of the last year or quarter. The BSC supplements financial measures with measures from three perspectives: customer, internal business, and innovation and learning.

The customer perspective examines how customers see the organization. The internal business perspective examines the activities, processes, and programs at which the organization must excel. The innovation and learning perspective, also referenced as the growth perspective, examines ways the organization can continue to improve and create value by looking at processes, procedures, and access to information to achieve the business strategies.

Used effectively, these three perspectives drive performance. For example, hypothetical Company XYZ developed a BSC that measures customer satisfaction. Their current assessment indicates a serious level of customer dissatisfaction. If not improved, lower sales will result. At the same time, however, the company's financial measures for the last two quarters indicate that sales are healthy. With only financial measures, management would conclude erroneously that the business is functioning well and they need not make changes. With the additional feedback from the customer measures, however, management knows that until recently they performed well, but that something is causing customer dissatisfaction. The company can investigate the cause of the results by interviewing customers and examining internal business measures. If the company is unable to improve customer satisfaction, eventually the result (lower sales) will appear in the financial measures.

The BSC provides organizations with a comprehensive view of the business and focuses management on the handful of measures that are the most critical. The BSC is more, however, than a collection of measures. If prepared properly, the BSC contains a unity of purpose that assures measures are directed to achieving a unified strategy. "Every measure selected for a BSC should be an element in a chain of cause-and-effect relationships, linkages, that communicates the meaning of the business unit's strategy to the organization." For example, do process improvements increase internal business efficiency and effectiveness? Do internal business improvements translate into improved customer service?

A good BSC incorporates a mix of outcome and output measures. Output measures communicate how the outcomes are to be achieved. They also provide an early indication about whether or not a strategy is being implemented successfully. Periodic reviews and performance monitoring tests the cause-and-effect relationships between measures and the appropriateness of the strategy.

Figure 10–1 illustrates the use of the BSC to link the vision and strategies of an SBU to critical performance measures via critical success factors. The BSC allows managers to examine the SBU from four important perspectives and to focus the strategic vision. The business unit puts the BSC to work by articulating goals for time, quality, and performance and service and then translates these goals into specific measures.

For each perspective, the SBU translates the vision and mission into the factors that will mean success. For the success factors to be critical, they must be necessary and sufficient for the SBU to succeed. Each critical success factor or objective needs to focus on a single topic and follow a verb-noun structure. For example, "Improve claims processing time (internal business perspective) by 'X' percent by 'Y' date." The more specific the objective, the easier it will be to develop performance measures. The less specific the objective, the more difficult it will be to develop performance measures.

Organizations are unique and will follow different paths to build the Balanced Scorecard. At Apple Computer and Advance Micro Devices, for example, a senior finance or business development executive, intimately familiar with the strategic thinking of the top management group, constructed the initial scorecard without extensive deliberations. The BSC provides federal agencies with a framework that serves as a performance measurement system and a strategic management system. This framework allows agencies to:

- Clarify and translate vision and strategy
- Communicate and link strategic objectives and measures
- Plan, set targets, and align strategic initiatives
- Enhance strategic feedback and learning

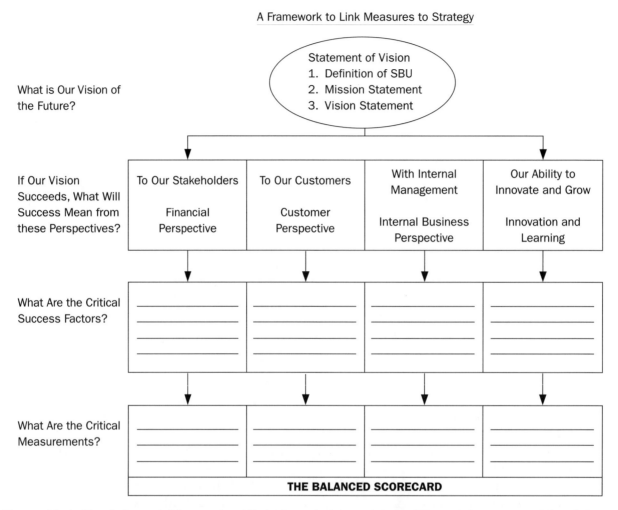

Figure 10–1. The Balanced Scorecard at Work. *Source:* Adapted from Office of Government Wide Policy, General Services Administration, "Eight Steps To Develop and Use Information Technology Performance Measures Effectively," Washington, D.C., GSA, December 1996.

Because federal agencies do not have the profit motive of private industry, the orientation of the BSC is different. For private industry, the financial perspective represents and assesses a company's profitability. The other perspectives represent and assess a company's future profitability. For government, the financial perspective represents the goals to control costs and to manage the budget. The customer perspective represents and assesses programs to serve taxpayers or society, other government agencies or other governments. The internal business and the innovation and learning perspectives represent and assess the government's ability to continually complete its mission.

The BSC addresses the contribution of IT to the business strategy in the learning and innovation perspective. The contribution includes improved access to information that may improve business processes, customer service and reduce operating costs. After the desired business outcomes and outputs are determined, the IT needs can be identified. A separate BSC is recommended for the IT support function to integrate and assess the IT services provided to the organization. Step 2 addresses the use of the BSC for the IT function and specific projects.

Clear strategic objectives, definitive critical success factors, and mission-level performance measures provide the best means to link IT projects to agency goals and objectives and ultimately agency accomplishments. Some believe that IT performance measures cannot be established until this has been done. Others believe that IT organizations must take the lead within their parent organizations to establish performance measures. Agencies may risk funding for their IT projects if they wait until critical success factors and mission-level measures are in place before developing IT performance measures. Whether the cart is before the horse or not, the experience gained from developing and using IT performance measures helps agencies develop more effective performance measures.

Agencies can identify information needs while developing strategic plans by having a member of the IT project management team (an individual who has extensive knowledge of the agency's programs and operations) involved in development of the strategic plans. At the least, grant a member access to the latest version of the plan. To identify information needs, agencies should define the following:

- Critical success factor(s) to be implemented
- Purpose and intended outcome
- Outputs needed to produce intended outcomes
- Users of the resulting product or service
- What the resulting product or service will accomplish
- Organizational units involved and their needs

IT professionals identify IT solutions that contribute to their agency's strategies and programs. They do this by exploring ways to apply technology to achieve one or more critical success factors. This requires an understanding of the organization, its structure and its operating environment. Successful IT project managers understand their agency's programs and processes and can describe how technology fosters improvement in agency business performance.

Linking IT projects to agency objectives requires involvement by senior management and consensus among stakeholders. Senior managers possess the broad perspective necessary for strategic planning. Stakeholders (e.g., managers, workers, support organizations, OMB, and Congress) have a vested interest in the project. They judge if linkage exists and to what degree it exists. The IT project manager identifies the stakeholders and works to obtain their agreement and support. The project manager faces the challenge of balancing the interests of internal and external stakeholders, which often differ.

Example of an IT Project Linked To Agency Goals and Objectives

Figure 10–2 shows how the Immigration and Naturalization Service (INS) linked its Integrated Computer Assisted Detection (ICAD) system performance measures to the agency's objectives. ICAD is the second generation of automated assisted detection systems used by the United States Border Patrol (USBP). With the installation of remote field sensors connected to Border Patrol communication facilities, ICAD displays remote sensor activity, processes incident (ticket) information, maintains the status of Border Patrol Agents in the field, provides access to state and national law enforcement services, and generates a variety of managerial reports. USBP management utilizes information that ICAD produces to make tactical decisions on the deployment of Border Patrol resources and strategic decisions on future Border Patrol operations.

The INS developed performance measures to show the effect of ICAD at the strategic, programmatic, and tactical levels of the organization. At the tactical level, the ICAD performance measures indicate the number of unlawful bordercrossers detected in two categories: migrant and smuggler. By increasing the effectiveness of the border patrol (programmatic level), ICAD contributes to achievement of the strategic goal to promote public safety by deterring criminal aliens. Figure 10–2 also shows the information INS uses to assess this goal.

Although the INS did not employ the BSC framework, they did use the following principles of the BSC: link IT to organization strategy; use a mix of short- and long-term measures; and select measures that have cause-and-effect relationships.

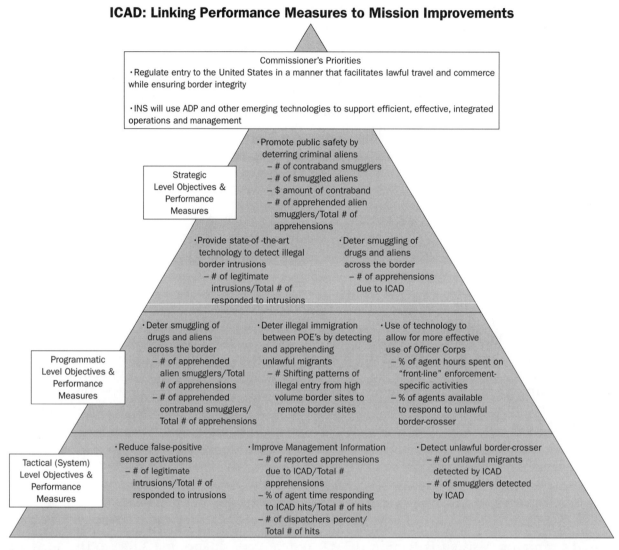

ICAD: Linking Performance Measures to Mission Improvements

Figure 10–2. The Immigration and Naturalization Service's Objectives and Measures for the Integrated Computer Assisted Detection System (ICAD). *Source:* Adapted from Office of Government Wide Policy, General Services Administration, "Eight Steps To Develop and Use Information Technology Performance Measures Effectively," Washington, D.C., GSA, December 1996.

Step 2 describes ways to determine what to measure and how to measure IT projects. It also provides an example of an agency IT measure and describes how to develop IT performance measures using the Balanced Scorecard.

Principles of Step 2

- Focus on the customer
- Select a few meaningful measures to concentrate on what's important

- Employ a combination of output and outcome measures
- Output measures assess efficiency; outcome measures assess effectiveness
- Use the Balanced Scorecard for a comprehensive view

Principles of Step 3

- Develop Baselines . . . they are essential to determine if performance improves
- Be sure baseline data is [sic] consistent with indicators chosen
- Use existing agency business reports where applicable

Principles of Step 4

- Value includes the IT project's return on investment and contribution to business priorities
- The major stakeholders determine the value of IT projects
- Select IT projects based upon value and risks

Principles of Step 5

- Focus on the customer
- Select data based upon availability, cost, and timeliness
- Make sure data is [sic] accurate . . . accuracy is more important than precision

Principles of Step 6

- Determine what worked . . . and what didn't
- Define the measures
- Prepare reports that track the results over time

Principles of Step 7

- Use results or no one will take measurement seriously
- Integrate results into business and technology domains
- Use results to improve performance, not evaluate people
- Hold individuals and teams accountable for managing for results

Principles of Step 8

- Communicate results . . . it's vital for continued support
- Share results in a manner that is useful and timely to:
  - Customers
  - Public
  - OMB
  - Congress . . .

Chapter 11

The Balanced Scorecard in Information Technology at the General Accounting Office

The General Accounting Office (GAO) has done some outstanding work in the area of information technology (IT) during the past few years. One of its better reports deals with the application of the BSC. The BSC application is in the larger area of measuring performance when investing in IT.

This application of the BSC is important because GAO has made the BSC an integral approach to measuring IT performance. In its five-practice continuum of performance management, the Balanced Scorecard is practice 2. The four areas of the Balanced Scorecard are:

1) Achieving the strategic needs of the enterprise
2) Satisfying the needs of individual customers
3) Addressing IT internal business performance
4) Addressing innovation and learning.

MEASURING PERFORMANCE AND DEMONSTRATING RESULTS OF INFORMATION TECHNOLOGY INVESTMENTS

The following material has been adapted from the U.S. General Accounting Office, Accounting and Information Management Division, *Executive Guide, Measuring Performance and Demonstrating Results of Information Technology Investments*, Washington, D.C., GAO, 1998, GAO/AIMD-98-89. A free copy of the report can be ordered from GAO by calling 202-512-6000.

Fundamental Practices: The Foundation of IT Performance Management

IT performance management and measures are considered **subsets** of overall performance management systems. In structuring an effective approach to performance management, it is also important to

- Differentiate between IT's impact on intermediate versus final program outcomes,
- Use a good balance of different kinds of IT measures,
- Understand that measures may differ by management tier within an organization, and
- Evaluate both the overall performance of the IT function within an organization and the outcomes for individual IT investments.

These concepts will be discussed in greater detail in subsequent sections of the guide.

Our approach suggests three primary practice areas that characterize IT performance management: *aligning* IT systems with agency missions, goals, and programs; *constructing* measures that determine how well IT is supporting strategic, customer, and internal business needs; and *implementing* performance measurement mechanisms at various decision-making levels within an organization.

Two supporting practice areas are important to keep the overall IT measurement process working: *Data collection and analysis capabilities,* which provide performance data that is [sic] accessible, reliable, and collected in the least burdensome manner. The benefit of effective automated data and management information systems is that performance information can be effectively and efficiently used to make strategic, managerial, and day-to-day operational decisions. In addition, a commitment to the concept of continuous improvement used for *strengthening the processes and practices being used to deliver IT products and services* is essential for maintaining effective IT organizations.

Figure 11–1 shows the generic model produced by our case study research on IT performance measurement.

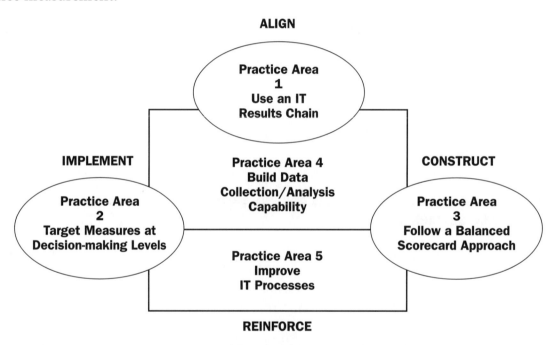

Figure 11–1. IT Performance Management Approach. *Source:* Adapted from U.S. General Accounting Office, Accounting and Information Management Division, *Executive Guide, Measuring Performance and Demonstrating Results of Information Technology Investments*, Washington, D.C., GAO, 1998, GAO/AIMD-98-89.

Practice Area 1: Follow an IT "Results Chain"

Leading organizations build and enforce a disciplined flow from goals to objectives to measures and individual accountability. They define specific goals, objectives, and measures, use a diversity of measure types, and describe how IT outputs and outcomes impact operational customer and enterprise (agency) program delivery requirements. The IT performance management system does not optimize individual customer results at the expense of an enterprise (agency) perspective.

Practice Area 2: Follow a Balanced Scorecard Approach

Leading organizations translate organizational strategy and IT performance expectations into a comprehensive view of both operational and strategic measures. Four generic goal areas include meeting the strategic needs of the enterprise, meeting the needs of individual operational customers, addressing internal IT business performance, and addressing ongoing IT innovation and learning.

Practice Area 3: Target Measures, Results, and Accountability at Different Decision-making Tiers

For the balanced scorecard areas, leading organizations match measures and performance results to various decision-making tiers or levels. These tiers include enterprise executives, senior to mid-level managers responsible for program or support units, and lower-level management running specific operations or projects. The organizations we studied document goals and measures in widely distributed IT performance improvement plans. Individual appraisals tie IT performance to incentives.

Practice Area 4: Build a Comprehensive Measure, Data Collection, and Analysis Capability

Leading organizations give considerable attention to base lining, benchmarking, and the collection and analysis of IT performance information. They use a variety of data collection and analysis tools and methods that serve to keep them informed but without imposing unnecessary reporting burdens. They also periodically review the appropriateness of their current measures.

Practice Area 5: Improve Performance of IT Business Processes To Better Support Mission Goals

In the leading organizations, IT performance improvement begins and ends with IT business processes. The organizations map their IT business processes and prioritize among those processes, which must be improved to support an enterprise and operational customers' business processes.

Practice Area 2: Follow a "Balanced Scorecard Approach"

PRACTICE AREA CHARACTERISTICS

1) Develop IT goals, objectives, and measures in operational and strategic areas
2) Focus on the most important "vital few" objectives and measures in four IT goal areas:
   - Achieving the strategic needs of the enterprise
   - Satisfying the needs of individual customers
   - Fulfilling IT internal business performance
   - Accomplishing IT innovation and learning

Practice Area Overview

A second best practice is to use a balanced scorecard approach to IT performance measurement. The approach attempts to create a measurement balance across the overall performance management framework. A balanced approach to measuring the contribution of IT to mission outcomes and performance improvement recognizes the broad impact of IT's supporting role. By measuring IT performance across four goal areas that are critical to overall IT success, the scorecard forces managers to consider measurement within the context of the whole organization. This limits the possibility of overemphasizing one area of measurement at the expense of others. In addition, measuring IT performance from different perspectives helps strengthen the analysis of intangible and tangible benefits attributable to technology.

In the four IT goal areas discussed in this section, we present three or four key objectives that were common among the organizations we examined. Corresponding to each objective we provide some sample measures that come from our case study research and from supporting literature. Our purpose is to illustrate possible types of measures, not to prescribe a definite list of measures that all organizations should be using. Some of the measures are very basic, but they are clearly related to the objectives. Also, many of the measures are percentages or ratios. This is important because successful organizations begin with good baseline data on performance and, therefore, can accurately measure progress against the baseline as they move forward.

In several of the organizations we studied, management is developing measures across key areas covering both long- and short-term strategies and activities. The Kaplan and Norton scorecard evaluates performance in four areas: financial (How does the organization look to shareholders?), customer (How do customers see performance?), internal business (At what must the organization excel?), and innovative and learning (Can the organization continue to improve and create value?).

In order to summarize the IT performance methods being used by the organizations we studied, we have adopted a balanced scorecard approach similar to the Kaplan and Norton framework. However, a balanced scorecard is just one approach available for agencies to adopt in conducting IT performance management and measurement. Other approaches such as the value management framework, critical success factor analysis, and information economics also offer useful IT performance measurement methodologies. Like other methodologies, a balanced scorecard approach translates organizational strategy into specific measurable objectives, operating from several key concepts:

- No single measure provides clear performance targets or places attention on critical mission areas,
- Goal, objective, and measure areas should give a comprehensive view of all levels of activities, from the project level to the strategic level,
- Limiting the number of measures used minimizes information overload, and
- A scorecard guards against optimizing one goal area at the expense of others.

Practice Area Characteristics

1. Develop IT Goals, Objectives, and Measures in Operational and Strategic Areas

For IT, measures cover a great diversity of value-added activities, including those for projects, a portfolio of applications, and infrastructure development. Organizations should know about success in all of them. As shown in Figure 11–2, an IT results chain can be translated into a scorecard framework that looks at goals, objectives, measures (tiered for various decision-making levels), and accountability in key goal areas. The key starting point in developing a balanced scorecard is the question of purpose from the IT results chain—"What is the current and future purpose of IT? Then to meet that purpose, the IT organization must must answer the goal question—"If we succeed, how will we differ?" in terms of specific goals.

The IT goals and objectives of the organizations we studied most often focused on the following:

- Customer commitments and satisfaction,
- Cycle and delivery time,
- Quality,
- Cost,
- Financial management,
- IT infrastructure availability,
- Internal IT operations,
- IT skill availability, and
- Customer business process support.

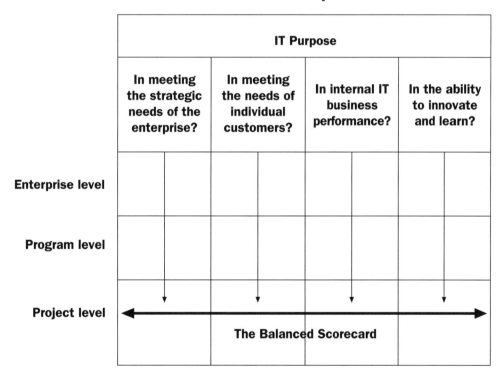

Figure 11-2. An IT Balanced Scorecard Approach. *Source:* Adapted from U.S. General Accounting Office, Accounting and Information Management Division, *Executive Guide, Measuring Performance and Demonstrating Results of Information Technology Investments*, Washington, D.C., GAO, 1998, GAO/AIMD-98-89.

For example, Motorola's Semiconductor Products Sector (SPS) focuses its goals and objectives on four areas: (1) delivering reliable products (quality environment, best-in-class staff, worldwide resource optimization, communication), (2) providing integrated IT solutions (integrated data and systems architecture, technology roadmap and migration planning, distributed computing effort), (3) building client partnerships (client involvement, lead the information technology community), and (4) achieving competitive advantage (prioritize the projects that benefit SPS, deploy resources for maximum impact, speed of execution).

We developed four balanced scorecard goal areas, objectives, and measures for IT that were among the most common across the organizations we studied. As such, the four goal areas illustrate an approximate consolidation of the performance management efforts of the organizations involved in our research. The four balanced scorecard goal areas are designed to measure how well IT is

- Achieving the strategic needs of the enterprise as a whole, in contrast to specific individual customers within the enterprise,
- Satisfying the needs of individual customers with IT products and services,
- Fulfilling internal IT business performance that delivers IT products and services for individual customers and the enterprise, and
- Accomplishing ongoing IT innovation and learning as IT grows and develops its skills and IT applications.

The first two goals address whether IT is providing the right products and services for the enterprise and individual customers. The latter two goal areas address how well IT is performing in its own capability to deliver those products and services. The strategic and customer perspectives are key for linking to mission planning requirements in the Results Act, the Chief Financial Officers Act, the Paperwork Reduction Act, and the Clinger-Cohen Act.

Managers in our case study organizations emphasized that "balance" does not necessarily mean "equality." Use of a balanced approach only means the consideration of several goal areas and the development of objectives and measures in each. For example, Kodak managers liked the balanced scorecard approach because it was a multivariable approach. Before using it, the IT organization was very cost conscious and tended to judge investments in new applications or skills largely from a cost perspective. The balanced scorecard examines short-term cost goals and potential business value in the context of various other nonfinancial operating parameters.

2. Focus on the "Vital Few" Objectives and Measures

Each leading organization customizes a set of measures appropriate for its organizational goals and, for IT, how IT fits into the enterprise's strategic direction and mission delivery plans. The organizations concentrate their IT performance management efforts on a vital few objectives and measures within the goal areas. The organizations did not severely limit the number of measures developed at the beginning. But, over time, and with experience, the organizations became more focused in the measures they used. However, use of a balanced scorecard approach gets rid of "safety net" measures which organizations often collect but do not use for decision-making, resource allocation, or oversight reporting purposes.

As is explained in the sections that follow, the measure examples illustrate the need for diversity. Within some of our case study organizations, similar measures are being used, but the measures remain under development, requiring more refinement and documentation. The measures presented here do not represent the full universe of what an organization might use. Also, in practice, the goal and objective areas may be more specific than those presented on the following pages. For example, one of our goal areas centers on the customer perspective. One objective of this goal area is customer satisfaction. In practice, an actual customer objective statement might be stated as "This fiscal year, at least 98 percent of customers will be satisfied with IT products, services, and processes." In short, the following sections discuss a general categorization of IT goals, objectives and sample measures.

Balanced Scorecard Goal Area 1: Achieving the Strategic Needs of the Enterprise

IT strategic measures are designed to evaluate the *aggregate* impact of IT investments on the organization. In short, these measures provide insights into impacts made by the organization's entire portfolio of IT investments.

This goal area focuses on ways to measure how IT supports the accomplishment of organizational strategies. The strategic perspective recognizes that in successful organizations, all components, including IT, must align with enterprise goals and directions.

When evaluating the impact of IT in terms of strategic needs, the following questions should be considered:

- How well integrated are our IT strategies with business needs?
- How well is the overall portfolio of IT investments being managed? Is IT spending in line with expectations?
- Are we consistently producing cost-effective results?
- Are we maximizing the business value and cost effectiveness of IT?

IT managers and staff often attempt to satisfy individual operational customers without a check against enterprise interests. Having this goal area prevents targeting IT efforts for individual operational customers, which may be very counter-productive to enterprise IT needs and expectations. Doing so is difficult, as one manager said, "It has been a cultural plan to look at [the company] as a whole versus maximizing for individual business partners. The reward and incentive systems are set up to emphasize that all senior managers must succeed together."

The four IT strategic enterprise objectives presented in Figure 11–3 reflect several key objective areas of the organizations we studied. These objectives cover enterprise strategic planning and goal accomplishment, enterprise management of the portfolio of IT applications, IT financial and investment performance, and use of IT resources across the enterprise.

The first objective in this goal area addresses how well IT plans and efforts reflect enterprise mission goals. This objective area assumes the enterprise has defined its mission goals and can make the clear link to how IT supports those goals. The sample measures capture the contribution of IT solutions and services, compare what was planned for IT benefits and IT strategies against what actually happened, and compare IT strategies and planning and enterprise strategies and planning. The overall measurement thrust is to make sure that enterprise mission goals direct IT activities.

The second objective, portfolio analysis and management, is a growing concern among the organizations we studied. Leading organizations want to make sure they have the right portfolio of IT applications either planned or in place that will enhance business or mission performance.

Kodak defines an application portfolio as a comprehensive inventory of computer applications that were developed or purchased to manage an organization's processes and information. The inventory contains detailed data relative to each application's size and characteristics, effectiveness in meeting business needs, potential for growth, and development and maintenance costs. The application portfolio forms the foundation for an overall IT investment strategy.

Objectives	Sample Measures
Enterprise	Percent mission improvements (cost, time, quality) attributable to IT mission goals solutions and services Percent planned IT benefits projected v. realized
Portfolio analysis and management	Percent IT portfolio reviewed and disposed Percent old applications retired Percent applications retirement plan achieved Percent reusable of core application modules Percent new IT investment v. total spending
Financial and investment performance	Percent and cost of services provided in-house v. industry standard IT budget as a percent of operational budget and compared to industry average Net present value, internal rate of return, return on investment, return on net assets
IT resource usage	Percent consolidated/shared resources across units Percent cross-unit shared databases and applications Percent hardware/software with interoperability capabilities

Figure 11–3. Balanced Scorecard—IT Strategic Measures. *Source:* Adapted from U.S. General Accounting Office, Accounting and Information Management Division, *Executive Guide, Measuring Performance and Demonstrating Results of Information Technology Investments*, Washington, D.C., GAO, 1998, GAO/AIMD-98-89.

Xerox has defined its IT inventory in a similar manner and made IT portfolio management a key objective area as part of its overall strategic enterprise strategies. As described in an earlier case study describing its IM2000 strategy, Xerox wanted to improve information management spending, deliver IT infrastructure renewal, and deliver process-driven IT solutions to customers. A key part of the overall IT strategy was to evaluate existing IT applications and determine how they supported, if at all, the IM2000 strategy. Xerox ran each of its existing applications through a rigorous analysis process, categorizing each into one of nine "disposition" categories ranging from stopping those of low usage and value to keeping others as corporate wide applications.

For Xerox, the IT portfolio strategy helps accomplish several performance goals. The strategy reduces unnecessary operational costs and increases support productivity; identifies and consolidates similar applications, and eliminates low value applications; identifies and retires legacy applications, data and infrastructure as new solutions are deployed; and identifies consolidation and sharing opportunities. The principle is to view application systems as corporate assets. (The Office of Management and Budget and GAO issued a guide, *Evaluating Information Technology Investments: A Practical Guide,* in November 1995 to assist federal agency and oversight staff in evaluating a portfolio of information technology investments in a similar manner. The approach is also an underlying feature of GAO's guide *Assessing Risks and Returns: A Guide for Evaluating Federal Agencies' IT Investment Decision-making* (GAO/AIMD-10.1.13, February 1997).)

The third objective in this goal area examines financial and investment performance. While the two objectives above cover mission goals and portfolio management, this objective addresses management of IT costs and returns. The sample measures capture costs in major IT financial categories such as hardware and software. They also provide information on the balance of spending between legacy and new development applications and between in-house and outsourced operations. Another sample measure compares the IT budget to the enterprise operational budget, and how that compares to industry standards.

Sample measures also look at the return on the IT investments, offering several different methodologies such as rate of return and net present value. Much of this information is traditionally benchmarked with other IT organizations of similar size and IT penetration. These measures are tied to customer and enterprise strategic perspectives to assess if scarce resources are being invested wisely. This is an especially important area in the federal government with the emphasis on cost reduction and the best possible use of existing resources.

Lastly, IT resource usage as an objective targets how well the organization can leverage and share its IT resources across the enterprise. The measures evaluate factors such as what resources can be shared, what has been consolidated, and employee access to computing services. From a strategic perspective, this objective recognizes the need for shared, enterprise wide applications and the use of an IT infrastructure and architecture for the entire organization.

Balanced Scorecard Goal Area 2: Satisfying the Needs of Individual Customers

IT customer measures are designed to measure the quality and cost effectiveness of IT products and services. When evaluating the impact of IT on customer satisfaction, the following questions should be considered:

- How well are business unit and IT staff integrated into IT systems development and acquisition projects?
- Are customers satisfied with the IT products and services being delivered?
- Are IT resources being used to support major process improvement efforts requiring information management strategies? If so, are the IT projects delivering the expected share of process improvement?

The purpose of the second goal area is to meet the needs of individual operational customers. The three objectives shown in Figure 11–4 capture the key objective areas we found in our research.

Objectives	Sample Measures
Customer partnership and involvement	Percent projects using integrated project teams Percent joint IT customer/supplier service-level agreements
Customer satisfaction	Percent customers satisfied with IT product delivery Percent customers satisfied with IT problem resolution Percent customers satisfied with IT maintenance and support Percent customers satisfied with IT training Percent products launched on time Percent service-level agreements met
Business process support	Percent IT solutions supporting process improvement projects Percent users covered by training to use new IT solutions Percent new users able to use applications unaided after initial training

Figure 11–4. Balanced Scorecard—IT Customer Measures. *Source:* Adapted from U.S. General Accounting Office, Accounting and Information Management Division, *Executive Guide, Measuring Performance and Demonstrating Results of Information Technology Investments*, Washington, D.C., GAO, 1998, GAO/AIMD-98-89.

Two of the objective areas, customer satisfaction and business process support, address direct IT support. Customers were especially interested in time, cost, quality, overall customer satisfaction, and business process support. One official we talked to said, "[Our IT organization] looks at the business process characteristics of our customers. IT personnel ask are there better ways to support product innovation and development? How does IT support that? The question is the effectiveness of IT in supporting business processes—not cranking out function points." A function point measures an IT application in terms of the amount of functionality it provides users. Function points count the information components of an application, such as external inputs and outputs and external interfaces.

The first objective area, customer partnership and involvement, stresses a mutual partnership between the IT organization and customers in developing the best possible IT products and services. The sample measures examine a variety of areas, ranging from cooperation and joint development to involvement in project management.

Customer satisfaction measures assess how well customers are satisfied with many IT activities. Sample measures also cover the accomplishment of system design requirements, complaints, problem resolution, error and defect rates, timeliness, and service-level agreement accomplishments.

The business process support objective area emphasizes the importance of business process improvement as organizations streamline and reengineer. Business process improvement is a central objective area for many of the organizations we studied. The sample measures capture how well IT supports business process improvement plans and process analysis. They also examine the adaptability of IT solutions, training for new IT solutions and the effectiveness of the training, and costs in moving applications to new hardware.

Balanced Scorecard Goal Area 3: Addressing IT Internal Business Performance

Internal IT business measures are designed to evaluate the operational effectiveness and efficiency of the IT organization itself. The ability of the IT shop to deliver quality products and services could have a direct impact on decisions to outsource IT functions. When evaluating internal IT business functions, the following questions should be considered:

- Are quality products delivered within general industry standards?
- Are quality products being delivered using accepted methods and tools?
- Is our infrastructure providing reliable support for business needs?
- Is the enterprise architecture being maintained and sustained?

One manager we interviewed said, "There are two dimensions of [IT] performance. One is the dominant or visible component—the use of IT in the context of [customer] business processes. The other is transparent—the functional excellence of IT." The first two goal areas stress the use of IT as it supports enterprise and operational customers. On a day-to-day basis, it is the functional excellence of IT internal business processes which delivers that support. Figure 11–5 shows four objective areas and sample measures we synthesized from our case study organizations and the general IT literature.

IT managers and staff, along with enterprise senior management, decide which of the many IT processes truly must excel for meeting customer and enterprise goals in the short and long term. For example, is the IT process for identifying the right technology for customer applications the best it can be? IT managers and staff set specific goals for improvement of internal IT business processes.

Objectives	Sample Measures
Applications development and maintenance	Number of function points delivered per labor hour Number of defects per 100 function points at user acceptance Number of critical defects per 100 function points in production Percent decrease in application software failures, problems Percent projects using standard methodology for systems analysis and design
Project performance	Percent projects on time, on budget Percent projects meeting functionality requirements Percent projects using standard methodology for systems analysis and design
Infrastructure availability	Percent computer availability Percent communications availability Percent applications availability On-line system availability
Enterprise architecture standards compliance	Number of variations from standards detected by review and audit per year Percent increase in systems using architecture Percent staff trained in relevant standards

Figure 11–5. Balanced Scorecard—IT Internal Business Measures. *Source:* Adapted from U.S. General Accounting Office, Accounting and Information Management Division, *Executive Guide, Measuring Performance and Demonstrating Results of Information Technology Investments*, Washington, D.C., GAO, 1998, GAO/AIMD-98-89.

The first objective covers IT's performance in developing and maintaining applications. The sample measures include dollars expended per function point, average application development cycle time, and cost. The second objective area examines the performance in delivering projects, capturing traditional measurements on project time, budget, functionality, and use of widely accepted methods and tools. Measures also capture backlogs in both development and enhancement or maintenance of applications.

The third objective area addresses IT infrastructure availability in a variety of areas, as well as response time and transactions. Many of the organizations we studied stressed the importance of infrastructure availability, an area totally transparent to the customer until something goes wrong. These measures keep managers on top of infrastructure performance where there is little tolerance for down time.

The last objective area covers architectural standards. IT architectures explicitly define common standards and rules for both data technology, as well as mapping key processes and information flows. A complete IT architecture should consist of both logical and technical components. The logical architecture provides the high-level description of the organization's mission, functional requirements, information requirements, systems components, and information flows among the components. The technical architecture defines the specific IT standards and rules that will be used to implement the logical architecture.

The measures assess how well IT is meeting set standards, most often developed for interconnectivity and interoperability and efficient IT support.

Many of the traditional IT measures fall into the internal business performance goal area, often focusing on the efficiency of computing and communications hardware and software.

The measures in this goal area frequently are used for individual manager and staff IT accountability, as described in a later practice.

Some of the organizations we studied were using the Software Engineering Institute's five-level capability maturity model to guide their IT process improvement efforts. The objective areas and measures are, in contrast to some of the other balanced scorecard areas, highly integrated. For example, project performance relies on effective applications development and maintenance.

Balanced Scorecard Goal Area 4: Addressing Innovation and Learning

Innovation and learning measures evaluate the IT organization's skill levels and capacity to consistently deliver quality results. This goal area recognizes that without the right people with the right skills using the right methodologies, IT performance will surely suffer. Measures in this goal area should be used to answer the following questions:

- Do we have the right skills and qualified staff to ensure quality results?
- Are we tracking the development of new technology important to our business/mission needs?
- Are we using recognized approaches and methods for building and managing IT projects?
- Are we providing our staff the proper tools, training, and incentives to perform their tasks?

The four objective areas shown in Figure 11–6 include workforce competency and development, advanced technology use, methodology currency, and employee satisfaction and retention.

Objectives	Sample Measures
Workforce competency and development	Percent staff trained in use of new technologies and techniques Percent staff professionally certified Percent IT management staff trained in management skills Percent IT budget devoted to training and staff development
Advanced technology use	Percent employees skilled in advanced technology applications Number of dollars available to support advanced technology skill development Percent projects using standard methodology for systems analysis and design
Methodology currency	Currency of application development methods used Percent employees skilled in advanced application development methods Percent projects developed using recognized methods and tools
Employee satisfaction and retention	Percent increase in systems using architecture Percent employee satisfaction with the capability of the existing technical and operating environment to support mission Percent employee turnover by function

Figure 11–6. Balanced Scorecard—IT Innovation and Learning Measures. *Source:* Adapted from U.S. General Accounting Office, Accounting and Information Management Division, *Executive Guide, Measuring Performance and Demonstrating Results of Information Technology Investments*, Washington, D.C., GAO, 1998, GAO/AIMD-98-89.

This goal area develops the continuous improvement aspect of IT activities. It speaks to capabilities of bringing new technologies to bear on customer problems, practicing the best methodologies, and retaining and developing the best employees. The first objective area stresses the importance of having a capable and competent workforce. In particular, the organizations we studied were very concerned with workforce competence and development. Key measures included training hours and skill development. Most were transitioning from core competencies in operations and maintenance to business process improvement and reengineering, new business solutions, and technical direction of applications development done by others.

The second and third objectives, advanced technology use and methodology currency, speak to the ability to recognize and deploy advanced technologies and methodologies in doing IT's work. The last objective, employee satisfaction and retention, measures how well employees themselves are satisfied with the quality of their work environment and general IT strategies and accomplishments.

How To Get Started

To begin developing a balanced scorecard approach for IT, organizations should

- Get agreement among business and IT management on the approach that will be used for developing IT-related performance measures,
- Using the agreed upon approach, define and develop the key goal areas and objectives for the IT organization,
- Develop a full set of measures in one or two priority IT goal areas, then expand out to other goal areas, and
- Test the performance measurement system and make revisions based upon initial lessons learned.

CHAPTER 12

The Balanced Scorecard in Procurement—Two Case Examples

There are two good examples of the application of the BSC in the procurement function. The first is the very broad and detailed work of the Procurement Executives' Association (PEA). The second example comes from the Department of Transportation.

PEA GUIDE TO THE BALANCED SCORECARD

The material that follows has been adapted from the Procurement Executives' Association, *Guide to a Balanced Scorecard: Performance Management Methodology: Moving from Performance Measurement to Performance Management.* The full guide can be accessed on the Web site of the Department of Energy (www.pr.doe.gov/pmmfinal.pdf).

Performance Management Strategy

This chapter sets forth the definitional baselines for performance measurement and performance management, provides a brief overview of the goals of a performance management system, and discusses a conceptual framework for performance measurement and management.

1. What Is Performance Management?

There are wide ranges of definitions for performance objective, performance goal, performance measure, performance measurement, and performance management. To frame the dialog and to move forward with a common baseline, certain key concepts need to be clearly defined and understood, such as:

Performance objective. This is a critical success factor in achieving the organization's mission, vision, and strategy, which if not achieved would likely result in a significant decrease in customer satisfaction, system performance, employee satisfaction or retention, or effective financial management.

Performance goal. A target level of activity expressed as a tangible measure, against which actual achievement can be compared.

Performance measure. A quantitative or qualitative characterization of performance.

Performance measurement. A process of assessing progress toward achieving predetermined goals, including information on the efficiency with which resources are transformed into goods and services (outputs), the quality of those outputs (how well they are delivered to clients and the extent to which clients are satisfied) and outcomes (the results of a program activity compared to its intended purpose), and the effectiveness of government operations in terms of their specific contributions to program objectives.

Performance management. The use of performance measurement information to effect positive change in organizational culture, systems, and processes, by helping to set agreed-upon performance goals, allocating and prioritizing resources, informing managers to either confirm or change current policy or program directions to meet those goals, and sharing results of performance in pursuing those goals.

Output measure. A calculation or recording of activity or effort that can be expressed in a quantitative or qualitative manner.

Outcome measure. An assessment of the results of a program compared to its intended purpose.

2. Performance Management System Goals

A leading-edge organization seeks to create an efficient and effective performance management system to:

- Translate agency vision into clear, measurable outcomes that define success, and that are shared throughout the agency and with customers and stakeholders;
- Provide a tool for assessing, managing, and improving the overall health and success of business systems;
- Continue to shift from prescriptive, audit- and compliance-based oversight to an ongoing, forward-looking strategic partnership involving agency headquarters and field components;
- Include measures of quality, cost, speed, customer service, and employee alignment, motivation, and skills to provide an in-depth, predictive performance management system; and
- Replace existing assessment models with a consistent approach to performance management.

3. The Balanced Scorecard Methodology

Leading organizations agree on the need for a structured methodology for using performance measurement information to help set agreed-upon performance goals, allocate and prioritize resources, inform managers to either confirm or change current policy or program direction to meet those goals, and report on the success in meeting those goals. To this end, in 1993 the Procurement Executives' Association (PEA) created the Performance Measurement Action Team (PMAT). Their task was to assess the state of the acquisition system, to identify a structured methodology to measure and improve acquisition performance, and to develop strategies for measuring the health of agency acquisition systems.

The PMAT found that organizations were using top-down management reviews to determine compliance with established process-oriented criteria and to certify the adequacy of the acquisition system. This method was found to lack a focus on the outcomes of the processes used and was largely ineffective in obtaining dramatic and sustained improvements in the quality of the operations.

The PMAT did extensive research and made site visits to leaders in performance measurement and management in an attempt to identify an assessment methodology appropriate for federal organizations. The model chosen was developed by Drs. David Norton and Robert Kaplan—the Balanced Scorecard (BSC) model. As modified by the PMAT, the measurement model identified critical success factors for acquisition systems, and developed performance measures within the four perspectives discussed below. Agencies which implemented the PMAT model utilized generic survey instruments and statistics obtained from the Federal Procurement Data System and other available data systems to determine the overall health of the system and how effectively it met its performance goals.

The work done by the PMAT has formed the foundation for the BSC methodology presented in this Guide. The lessons learned, and the best practices and strategies resulting from the PMAT experience, were used to create an expanded and enhanced BSC model. The PEA believes this revised methodology to be the best for deploying an organization's strategic direction, communicating its expectations, and measuring its progress toward agreed-to objectives. Additionally, a 1998 study by the Gartner Group found that "at least 40% of Fortune 1000 companies will implement a new management philosophy . . . the Balanced Scorecard . . . by the year 2000."

The BSC presented in this Guidebook is a conceptual framework for translating an organization's vision into a set of performance indicators distributed among four perspectives: financial, customer, internal business processes, and learning and growth. Some indicators are maintained to measure an organization's progress toward achieving its vision; other indicators are maintained to measure the long-term drivers of success. Through the balanced scorecard, an organization monitors both its current performance (finance, customer satisfaction, and business process results) and its efforts to improve processes, motivate and educate employees, and enhance information systems—its ability to learn and improve.

4. The Four Perspectives of the Balanced Scorecard

Financial. In the government arena, the "financial" perspective differs from that of the traditional private sector. Private sector financial objectives generally represent clear long-range targets for profit-seeking organizations, operating in a purely commercial environment. Financial considerations for public organizations have an enabling or a constraining role, but will rarely be the primary objective for business systems. Success for public organizations should be measured by how effectively and efficiently they meet the needs of their constituencies. Therefore, in the government, the financial perspective emphasizes cost efficiency, i.e., the ability to deliver maximum value to the customer.

Customer. This perspective captures the ability of the organization to provide quality goods and services, the effectiveness of their delivery, and overall customer service and satisfaction. In the governmental model, the principal driver of performance is different than in the strictly commercial environment; namely, customers and stakeholders take preeminence over financial results. In general, public organizations have a different, perhaps greater, stewardship/fiduciary responsibility and focus than do private sector entities.

Internal business processes. This perspective focuses on the internal business results that lead to financial success and satisfied customers. To meet organizational objectives and customers' expectations, organizations must identify the key business processes at which they must excel. Key processes are monitored to ensure that outcomes will be satisfactory. Internal business processes are the mechanisms through which performance expectations are achieved.

Learning and growth. This perspective looks at the ability of employees, the quality of information systems, and the effects of organizational alignment in supporting accomplishment of organizational goals. Processes will only succeed if adequately skilled and motivated employees, supplied with accurate and timely information, are driving them. This perspective takes on increased importance in organizations, like those of the PEA members, that are undergoing radical change. In order to meet changing requirements and customer expectations, employees may be asked to take on dramatically new responsibilities, and may require skills, capabilities, technologies, and organizational designs that were not available before.

Figure 12–1 visually depicts the global BSC framework. . . .

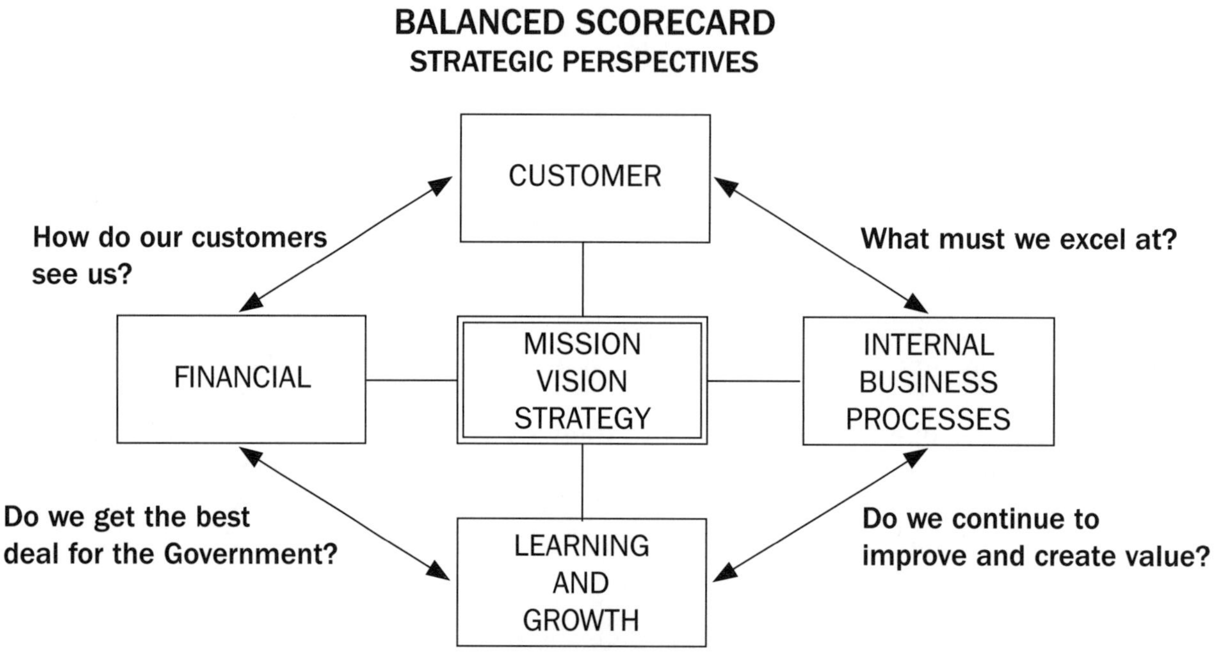

BALANCED SCORECARD
STRATEGIC PERSPECTIVES

Figure 12–1. The Global BSC Framework. *Source:* Adapted from Procurement Executives' Association, *Guide to a Balanced Scorecard: Performance Management Methodology: Moving from Performance Measurement to Performance Management,* www.pr.doe.gov/pmmfinal.pdf.

5. Implementing a Balanced Scorecard
A. Collaborative efforts. To realize the full benefits of the BSC, the PEA encourages the adoption of the BSC for all key agency functions.

- Implementing the BSC agency-wide will provide: (1) a common methodology and coordinated framework for all agency performance measurement efforts; (2) a common "language" for agency managers; (3) a common basis for understanding measurement results; and (4) an integrated picture of the agency overall.
- While implementing the acquisition BSC is an important first step, helping agencies to develop BSCs for additional functions (e.g., program, human resources, finance, IT) will strengthen the link among the acquisition system, those additional functions, and agency missions and goals. This will highlight how performance improvement initiatives in one area positively or negatively affect performance in another area. Also, this will promote cross-functional coordination of improvement efforts and help break down "stovepipes" in the agency.
- Acquisition executives may serve as advocates to promote the benefits of BSC agency-wide by advertising successful improvement efforts, and by discussing the BSC methodology in meetings with the Secretary, Administrator, or senior-level managers in other functional areas.
- The BSC will provide sound data on which to base business decisions, from allocation of available resources to future direction. This will enable the agency to manage its activities and its resources more effectively. For example, the BSC could form a common basis to support a business case for more resources.
- While we believe the Procurement Executive should promote the BSC's benefits and encourage its adoption beyond the acquisition realm, an agency can benefit even if it ultimately decides to adopt the BSC only for its acquisition function. The four perspec-

tives provide a useful framework for analyzing and understanding how acquisition supports accomplishment of the agency's mission. The information gained will help the agency assess how its acquisition system is performing, whether it is meeting its objectives, and whether it is moving in the direction envisioned in the FAR guiding principles. *As the key leader for the acquisition BSC, the Procurement Executive has a critical role in ensuring its successful implementation and use, and is responsible for setting into motion the steps recommended in this Guide.*

B. Pathway to success. A federal agency can take several steps to encourage support for BSC activities or any performance measurement and improvement efforts within its organization:

1. **Make a commitment at all levels—especially at the top level.** Research clearly shows that strong leadership is paramount in creating a positive organizational climate for nurturing performance improvements. Senior management leadership is vital throughout the performance measurement and improvement process. By senior management, we mean the organizational level that can realistically foster cross-functional, mission-oriented performance improvements—from senior operating or functional managers in the various acquisition and program offices throughout a federal agency, to the Secretary or Administrator of the agency. Senior management should have frequent formal and informal meetings with employees and managers to show support for improvement efforts and implementation initiatives. Also, they should frequently review progress and the results of improvement efforts.

2. **Develop organizational goals.** Goals need to be specified and publicized to provide focus and direction to the organization. Vision Statements and Strategic/Tactical Plans (including systematic ways to evaluate performance) are important for methodically planning acquisition performance improvements. To be meaningful, they must include measurable objectives along with realistic timetables for their achievement. For acquisition measures, it may be appropriate to use or build upon the performance principles and standards set forth in the Federal Acquisition Regulation (FAR) Subpart 1.102 to develop goals, whether they are stand-alone goals or a subset of larger, overarching organizational goals. Providing guidance on the best way to link acquisition goals to annual, mission-oriented GPRA performance plans is also essential. This will demonstrate that the agency is serious about acquisition improvement initiatives.

3. **Offer training in improvement techniques.** Training should be provided to appropriate personnel to help them properly make process improvements. The scope of training should include the operation of integrated project improvement teams; the role employees play in exercising sound business judgment, and the specific techniques for making process improvements (e.g., flowcharts, benchmarking, cause-and-effect diagrams, etc.). Comprehensive training is needed to expand employees' technical capabilities and to achieve "buy-in" for undertaking meaningful improvement efforts. Use of facilitators can provide "just-in-time" training to members of process action teams.

4. **Establish a reward and recognition system to foster performance improvements.** In our view, agencies should tie any reward and recognition system to performance improvement as measured by the acquisition BSC. Thus, employee incentives will tend to reinforce the organizational objectives being measured by the acquisition BSC. While handing out rewards to individual employees has its place, group reward and recognition systems are also needed to encourage integrated, cross-functional teams of employees, customers and managers to undertake acquisition performance improvement. Agencies may wish to consult with OPM and OMB for suggestions on the most suitable types of rewards and recognition (e.g., plaques, bonuses, etc.).

5. **Break down organizational barriers.** To overcome unfounded fears about the perceived adverse effects of performance measurement and improvement, we believe that the official uses of the acquisition BSC need to be spelled out to employees and managers. For example, it might be useful to invite representatives from the National Partnership for Reinventing Government (formerly known as the National Performance Review), Office of Federal Procurement Policy, the PEA Team, and the agency's own senior-level management to speak to key agency personnel on the purpose of undertaking customer surveys, performance measurement, and process improvement. These officials could explain that the performance measurement data is to be used to promote self-assessment, self-improvement, progress in acquisition reform, linkage to overall mission goals, and collaborative cross-agency benchmarking—not to take reprisals against individuals or organizations. Also, we recommend presentation of "success stories" that demonstrate the non-threatening nature of the BSC methodology, including how an agency can target areas most in need of improvement, benchmark against best-in-class organizations, and form integrated project teams to undertake performance improvements. Stakeholders must be shown that a cooperative effort toward performance improvement is the most appropriate course of action—that supporting the BSC is in their best interest.

6. **Coordinate headquarters and field office responsibilities.** Implementation should be a collaborative effort between an agency's lead corporate office (such as an acquisition management office at HQ) and its local (or field) offices. The offices should jointly decide on their respective roles and responsibilities relative to the BSC. In most cases, the lead corporate office is in the best position to provide leadership, oversight, and a well-defined methodology. The assignment of other roles and responsibilities will differ based on what is appropriate for the offices' circumstances, such as:

   • How centralized or decentralized the offices are.
   • The extent to which data are collected from a centralized information system or from local databases.
   • The extent to which surveys are conducted centrally or locally.

   Some PEA agencies have found that local acquisition offices are best suited for implementing the actual assessment process by generating quantitative data from appropriate sources, and by conducting surveys to obtain the necessary feedback for making procurement system improvements. The lead corporate office provides local offices the tools, training, software programs, and guidance they need to compile and examine their own results. This might include computer templates that help select survey samples, generate mailing labels, enter survey data, track survey data, and analyze survey data. The local offices also provide advice on accessing and compiling quantitative Management Information System (MIS) data; while the lead office encourages the use of existing quantitative data systems for multiple performance measurement purposes. Under this model, in partnership with the local offices, the lead corporate office:

   • Assumes a leadership role in developing and refining the survey instruments to be used.
   • Prepares generic cover letters.
   • Facilitates the conduct of surveys at the local offices.
   • Fosters local improvement initiatives (including benchmarking) resulting from the survey efforts.
   • Monitors response rates, compliance with the required statistical methodology, and overall survey administration progress.

With a clearly defined methodology in hand, the local procurement offices in these agencies:

- Develop their own mailing lists.
- Select their own samples.
- Print and mail the surveys.
- Compile their own survey data.
- Track and analyze the office-unique survey results.
- Generate their own management information system quantitative data.

We recommend that there be an agreement among the lead corporate office and local offices to use a set of common measures, instruments, supporting computer templates and improvement strategies in line with PEA tenets. This agreement should rest firmly on a cooperative relationship between the corporate lead office and the local offices, in which both have worked closely together to design and build their BSC-based performance measurement and improvement system. In some cases, the agreement may give local procurement offices the discretion to use additional, office-specific measures.

C. Other key steps. What follows are some additional approaches that will help in successfully implementing a performance measurement and improvement system:

- **Demonstrate a clear need for improvement.** If you cannot demonstrate a genuine need to improve the organization, failure is a virtual certainty.
- **Make realistic initial attempts at implementation.** If your initial attempts are too aggressive, the resulting lack of organizational "buy-in" will limit your chance of success. Likewise, if implementation is too slow, you may not achieve the necessary organizational momentum to bring the BSC to fruition.
- **Integrate the scorecard into the organization.** Incorporating performance measurement and improvement into your existing management structure, rather than treating it as a separate program, will greatly increase the BSC's long-term viability.
- **Change the corporate culture.** To achieve long-term success, it is imperative that the organizational culture evolve to the point where it cultivates performance improvement as a continuous effort. Viewing performance improvement as a one-time event is a recipe for failure.
- **Institutionalize the process.** Creating, leveraging, sharing, enhancing, managing, and documenting BSC knowledge will provide critical "corporate continuity" in this area. A knowledge repository will help to minimize the loss of institutional performance management knowledge that may result from retirements, transfers, promotions, etc. . . .

How To Establish Performance Measures

This chapter provides a methodology for establishing performance measures within the four perspectives of the balanced scorecard approach and for ensuring that the measures fit within an overall management approach. . . .

How can an organization establish performance measures that make sense? There are many variations to the theme. As indicated earlier, we found the approach presented by Kaplan and Norton to be the most effective, particularly for ensuring that measures relate to the specific vision and mission of the organization. This approach is only one of many. Which method you use will depend on your organization, its culture, and its mission.

1. Define Organizational Vision, Mission, and Strategy

The BSC methodology, as with most performance management methodologies, requires the creation of a vision, mission statement, and strategy for the organization. This ensures that the performance measures developed in each perspective support accomplishment of the organization's strategic objectives. It also helps employees visualize and understand the links between the performance measures and successful accomplishment of strategic goals.

The key, as pointed out by Kaplan and Norton, is to first identify where you want the organization to be in the near future. Set a vision—a vision that seems somewhat out of reach. In this way, "[t]he Balanced Scorecard . . . provides managers with the instrumentation they need to navigate to future competitive success." (Kaplan and Norton)

2. Develop Performance Objectives, Measures, and Goals

Next, it is essential to identify what the organization must do well (i.e., the performance objectives) in order to attain the identified vision. For each objective that must be performed well, it is necessary to identify measures and set goals covering a reasonable period of time (e.g., three to five years). Sounds simple, however, many variables impact how long this exercise will take. The first, and most significant, variable is how many people are employed in the organization and the extent to which they will be involved in setting the vision, mission, measures, and goals.

The BSC translates an organization's vision into a set of performance objectives distributed among four perspectives: Financial, Customer, Internal Business Processes, and Learning and Growth. Some objectives are maintained to measure an organization's progress toward achieving its vision. Other objectives are maintained to measure the long-term drivers of success. Through the use of the BSC, an organization monitors both its current performance (financial, customer satisfaction, and business process results) and its efforts to improve processes, motivate and educate employees, and enhance information systems—its ability to learn and improve. Figure 12–2 . . . provides matrices used in the BSC methodology to help develop objectives and measures. The matrices are relatively straightforward and easy to understand. However, developing the contents of each matrix is the hard part.

When creating performance measures, it is important to ensure that they link directly to the strategic vision of the organization. The measures must focus on the outcomes necessary to achieve the organizational vision and the objectives of the strategic plan. When drafting measures and setting goals, ask whether or not achievement of the identified goals will help achieve the organizational vision.

Each objective within a perspective should be supported by at least one measure that will indicate an organization's performance against that objective. Define measures precisely, including the population to be measured, the method of measurement, the data source, and the time period for the measurement. If a quantitative measure is feasible and realistic, then its use should be encouraged.

When developing measures, it is important to include a mix of quantitative and qualitative measures. Quantitative measures provide more objectivity than qualitative measures. They may help to justify critical management decisions on resource allocation (e.g., budget and staffing) or systems improvement. An agency should first identify any available quantitative data and consider how it can support the objectives and measures incorporated in the BSC. Qualitative measures involve matters of perception, and therefore of subjectivity. Nevertheless, they are an integral part of the BSC methodology. Judgments based on the experience of customers, employees, managers, and contractors offer important insights into acquisition performance and results.

For example, while an agency will usually need surveys to gauge some elements of customer satisfaction such as timeliness of service, process-oriented measures such as acquisi-

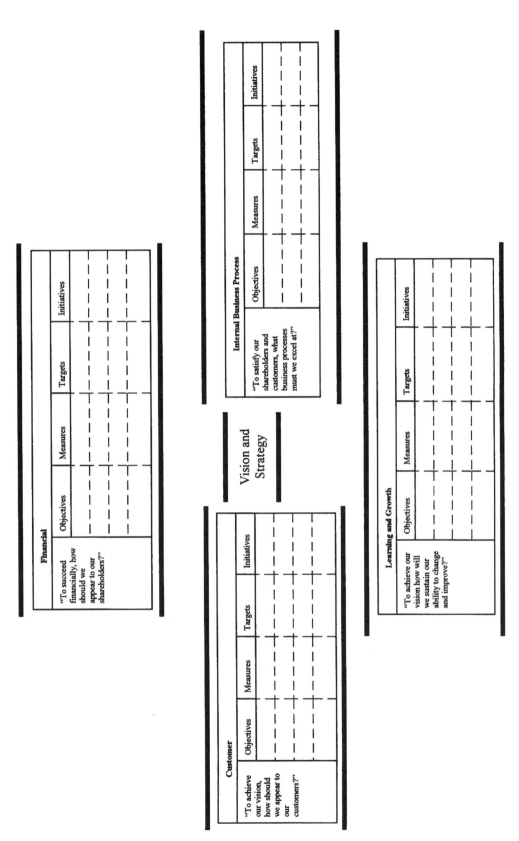

Figure 12–2. Matrices Used in the Balanced Scorecard Methodology. *Source: Adapted from Procurement Executives' Association, Guide to a Balanced Scorecard: Performance Management Methodology: Moving from Performance Measurement to Performance Management, www.pr.doe.gov/ pmmfinal.pdf.*

tion lead time or contract delivery time may be used as supplemental quantitative indicators—they help explain the underlying reasons for survey performance results. Achieving a balance among quantitative and qualitative factors (as well as among process-oriented and results-driven measures) is crucial in developing a valid BSC methodology.

The evolution of all performance measurements should begin with an organization's Strategic Plan. Figure 12–3, "Integrating Performance Measurement with Other Business Strategies," is a model which depicts a timeline for the business strategies/processes and strategic events that could occur within an organization, and the integration of performance measurement (in this case, acquisition performance measurement) within the process. A synopsis of each follows:

- **Strategic plan.** The Strategic Plan is a five-year plan that extends (in the model) from FY 1997 to FY 2002. It is the one document that sets forth the overall direction, vision, and mission of the organization and recognizes the requirement to set performance goals and to identify measures to gauge progress toward these goals.
- **Performance plan.** To accomplish the Strategic Plan, an annual Performance Plan is developed. This plan defines the measures, activities, and goals that, when taken together, indicate how well the organization's overall goals are being achieved.
- **Budget process.** The budget defines the resources needed to accomplish the strategic goals. Within this process, senior acquisition managers (e.g., procurement heads) develop an acquisition budget strategy, which is an integral step to strengthening budgetary requests and obtaining the resources to meet strategic planning and performance goals.
- **Procurement performance measurement plan.** Following down the strategic planning process, more and more refined performance measures are utilized. This plan can be the document that provides the specific link to the Strategic and Performance Plans. The foundation of the Procurement Performance Measurement Plan stems from the goals, objectives, and measures of the Strategic and Performance Plans.

Many models exist for translating the performance measures of the organization into an individual's performance plan. One of our participating agencies is employing the model shown in Figures 12–4 and 12–5. Figure 12–4, "Performance Management Framework," depicts how strategic initiatives can flow from the agency strategic plan down to an acquisition organization's strategies and then into objectives, measures, targets, and initiatives. This figure becomes the foundation for developing performance plans. Figure 12–5, "Employee Performance Management," shows how the performance measures, using the BSC framework, can be developed following the flow-down of strategic guidance from the agency level down to the individual acquisition official performance plan level. By tying an individual's performance appraisal to the organization's strategic goals, it helps employees understand the vision, mission, and goals of the organization, and motivates employees to work as a team to support initiatives that directly relate to the corporate goals by rewarding them for organizational accomplishments and not just individual achievements.

3. Evolve with Experience

Finally, it takes time to establish measures, but it is also important to recognize that they might not be perfect the first time. Performance management is an evolutionary process that requires adjustments as experience is gained in the use of performance measures. . . .

INTEGRATING PERFORMANCE MEASUREMENT WITH OTHER BUSINESS STRATEGIES
(A MODEL)

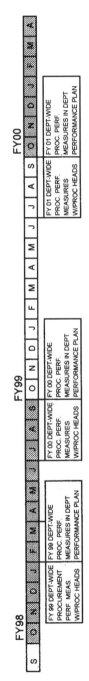

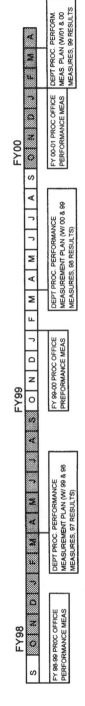

Figure 12–3. Integrating Performance Measurement with Other Business Strategies: A Model. *Source:* Adapted from Procurement Executives' Association, *Guide to a Balanced Scorecard: Performance Management Methodology: Moving from Performance Measurement to Performance Management,* www.pr.doe.gov/pmmfinal.pdf.

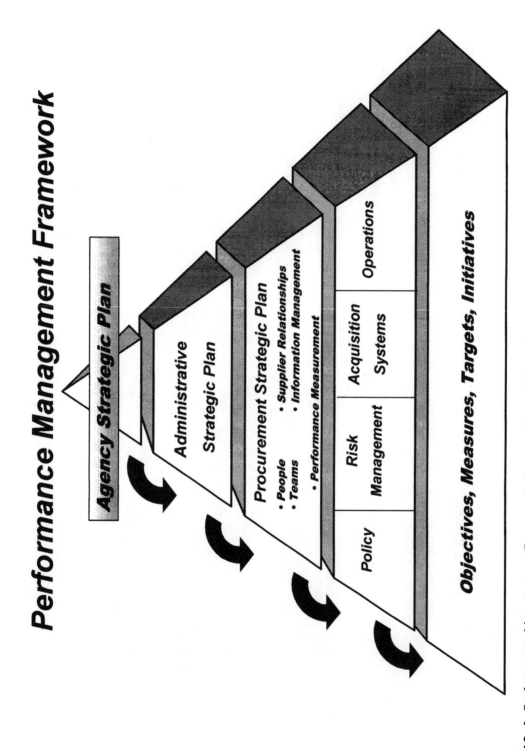

Figure 12–4. Performance Management Framework. *Source:* Adapted from Procurement Executives' Association, *Guide to a Balanced Scorecard: Performance Management Methodology: Moving from Performance Measurement to Performance Management,* www.pr.doe.gov/pmmfinal.pdf.

Employee Performance Management

AGENCY STRATEGIC PLAN

Strategic Priorities:
-

Programs	Measures

ADMINISTRATIVE STRATEGIC PLAN

Strategic Priorities:
- Risk Management
- Integrated Policy and Planning
- Development and Diversity

- Information Technology
- Financial Management
- Customer Service

Responsibilities	Measures

PROCUREMENT EXECUTIVE PERFORMANCE PLAN

Strategic Priorities:
- Customer Satisfaction
- Effective Service Partnership
- Minimize Administrative Cost

- Acquisition Excellence
- Information for Strategic Decision Making
- Quality Workforce

Customer	Financial	Internal Business Process	Learning and Growth
- % Customer Satisfaction w/ Timeliness - % Customer Satisfaction w/ Quality - % Customer Satisfaction w/ responsiveness, cooperation, and communication to meet mission	- Cost to Spend Ratio - Cost avoidance through use of purchase cards - Prompt payment interest paid vs. total $ disbursed	- Ratio of protest upheld at GAO and COFC - # of actions using electronic commerce - % achievement of Socio-economic goals - % Competitive procurement of total procurements	- Extent of reliable management information - % of employees meeting mandatory standards - % of employees satisfied with the work environment - % of employees satisfied with the professionalism, culture, values and empowerment

Figure 12–5. Employee Performance Management. Source: Adapted from Procurement Executives' Association, *Guide to a Balanced Scorecard: Performance Management Methodology: Moving from Performance Measurement to Performance Management,* www.pr.doe.gov/pmmfinal.pdf.

Data Collection

In Chapters Three and Four, we identified a variety of measures that may be used in an acquisition balanced scorecard. Some of the measures fall within the purview of quantitative metrics, while others are of a more qualitative nature. In this chapter, we discuss the key ground rules for collecting reliable performance data to track these quantitative and qualitative measures.

1. Basic Principles

Whether data are quantitative or qualitative, applying the two basic data collection principles identified below will help an agency to obtain reliable data in the most efficient manner. Using these principles, an agency may find synergies between existing, separate systems. Defining links where data collection serves multiple purposes can improve efficiency, support partnerships among organizations, and provide a framework for future system improvements.

A. Use existing data sources to the extent feasible. Many agency management information systems already collect reliable quantitative data, which are useful for acquisition performance measures; and agencies likely have large investments in these systems. These systems include financial, personnel, and administrative systems, as well as contractual information systems. Contractual information systems encompass agency feeder systems to the FPDS, as well as electronic commerce databases (e.g., GSA's Electronic Commerce Online Statistics Reporting System).

For example, the agency may already track measures on workforce training and education as part of a contracting officer warrant program. Also, some data necessary for an acquisition measure may be regularly captured and reported through a management information system that supports another agency function, such as finance or small business. An agency's existing quantitative data typically cover a broad spectrum—from workforce quality, procurement lead-time, and extent of compliance with socioeconomic goals to the use of electronic commerce, contract protest records, and competition statistics.

Moreover, qualitative data from existing acquisition surveys may be used to support BSC efforts. Some agencies have designed and already use acquisition-specific surveys. Much of the data collected by those surveys will be useful for the BSC with little or no change. In some cases, other agency survey instruments collect acquisition-related data. For example, an agency-wide employee survey may collect information useful for the learning and growth element if the acquisition-related information can be segregated. The agency should avoid duplicative surveys and maximize the use of results from a minimum number of surveys.

Data in an automated system should be used directly from that system instead of having to re-enter it into a separate system that supports the BSC. Using existing data sources for multiple reporting purposes improves data reliability by minimizing the potential for errors in repetitive data entry. It also minimizes the burden of data collection and training, thereby promoting greater acceptance of the BSC. Of course, agencies need to ensure that all users have a common understanding of each shared data element.

B. Automate data collection where possible. While many agencies have management information systems that are partially automated, we encourage the expanded use of automation to compile important quantitative data, where efficient and cost-effective. Moreover, as technology evolves, we expect more and more surveys to be administered electronically (e.g., using e-mail hyper-linked to the Web) with automated qualitative survey results going directly into applications that gauge performance. Automation will tend to save time, reduce error rates, and obviate the need for separate data entry and verification.

However, to ensure the validity of automated surveys, data reliability standards must still be maintained, survey recipients must have equal access to relevant electronic media (e.g., e-mail; Web, etc.), and the corporate culture must be technologically sophisticated enough to make survey participants willing to apply this new medium to surveys. For example, if an agency's contractors were to receive an electronic version of a survey; print it in hard copy; and return the completed hard-copy survey by mail (instead of completing and returning the survey on-line) the advantage of using the automated process would be lessened. More important, if contractors are not receptive to an electronic survey process, they may simply delete the initial automated survey transmission—leading to poor response rates. In light of these factors, we recommend that automation be used on a selective basis for internal surveys (i.e., employee, customer, or manager surveys) and only sparingly for external (contractor/vendor) surveys. In addition, e-mail alert notices and reminders will be instrumental in achieving adequate response rates, especially for automated external surveys.

2. Survey Methodology

If the basic principles identified above are followed, agencies will be able to compile management information for quantitative metrics in a rather straightforward fashion. However, since collecting qualitative data is much more demanding, you may wish to avail yourselves of the following overview of survey methodology to help you maintain data integrity.

A. Survey populations & instruments. . . . As explained in Chapter Four, the PEA has decided to collect core, common performance data on a variety of measures—some of which are compiled using surveys. The sample survey instruments address core, common performance objectives (e.g., Customer Satisfaction, Employee Satisfaction, etc.). They also build upon the survey instruments developed under the original PMAT model, are basically equivalent to one another in content, and lay a firm, consistent foundation for cross-agency benchmarking. However, each participating agency retains the flexibility to tailor the survey instruments to meet its own needs.

The sample survey instruments address different types of measures, and involve different types of participants. Under the "Learning and Growth" perspective, the Procurement Employee Survey addresses the core measures of Quality Work Environment and Executive Leadership. It reflects questions the agency should ask office employees, supervisors, and managers. Under the "Customer" perspective, the Procurement Customer Survey targets the core measures of Timeliness, Service/Partnership, and Quality. It reflects questions the agency should ask customers internal to the agency who use items or services delivered by contract (direct internal customers). The questions also apply to customers outside the agency who generate requirements (direct external customers).

In addition, some agencies use a Self-Assessment "survey" to capture qualitative data for the core performance objective of "Information Availability for Strategic Decision-Making" under the "Learning & Growth" perspective, as well as other measures such as Mission Goals or Contract Administration. (It is worth noting that some agencies also include optional quantitative metrics under the Self-Assessment umbrella). The self-assessment survey questions are for contracting office managers, who may call upon lower level supervisors for their contributions. Also, some agencies use a Contractor/Vendor Survey in order to better understand their vendors' (i.e., industry partners') perspective about the efficiency, timeliness, quality, and cooperation of agency acquisition and program offices—thus promoting the incorporation of best industry standards into agency acquisition practices.

B. Survey design. Surveys should be designed in accordance with current research techniques. For example, survey instruments should be brief, with only very basic information requested to measure satisfaction and to obtain feedback on areas that may require improvement. Agencies would do well to: formulate simple and direct questions; avoid open-ended questions; make the questionnaire answerable within 15 minutes; group questions into categories for ease of response; assure anonymous responses; present the questions in a user-friendly booklet form; and pre-test the questionnaire to ensure minimal respondent burden and facilitate as high a response rate as possible. Pre-testing the survey instruments will allow agencies to eliminate or revise questions as necessary, add material that the representative respondents strongly believe should be included, and improve the overall quality and utility of the instruments.

Using a Strongly Disagree to Strongly Agree (or equivalent) rating scale, examples of simple and direct survey questions might include the following:

- "My work schedule is flexible." [Quality Work Environment, under Employee Survey]
- "Customers respect my procurement office." [Executive Leadership, under Employee Survey]
- "Obtains products/services when I need them." [Timeliness, under Customer Survey]
- "Deals with me in a courteous, business-like manner." [Service/Partnership, under Customer Survey]
- "Obtains high-quality products/services." [Quality, under Customer Survey]

Incorporating background questions (e.g., business category; type of product or service) will allow for later multivariate statistical analysis so that an agency may assess whether differences in categories of respondents' backgrounds help explain differences in responses to individual questions (e.g., whether contractor satisfaction varies by type of business organization). This information will help agencies to better target opportunities for acquisition system improvements. Moreover, it is recommended that a "comments" section be added at the very end of the survey for obtaining respondents' observations on good practices and procedures, descriptions of problem areas, and recommendations for solving those problems. A "comments" section often contributes to receiving higher response rates.

C. Statistical survey methodology. Survey procedures are needed to make sure that agencies obtain sound statistical data. Reliable data depend heavily on selecting representative survey participants, targeting the proper sample size, and obtaining reasonably high response rates. Thus, the methodology that follows is designed to ensure that individual agencies conduct the BSC surveys according to accepted statistical standards. Since developing and implementing statistical survey procedures is an exacting discipline, please bear in mind that some of the terminology used below may get somewhat technical at times. You may wish to consult with a trusted statistician to guide you through any unfamiliar statistical terrain.

In general, each participating agency should plan to take a 50 percent sample for populations of 1,000 or fewer—based on a hypergeometric distribution—to achieve precision of plus or minus 3 percent at the 95 percent confidence level. [Unlike a normal distribution, a hypergeometric distribution applies to very small populations.] For example, if we receive survey results indicating that 58 percent of customer survey participants strongly agree that some acquisition function is performed well, then we can say that between 55 percent and 61 percent of customers feel that way—58 percent plus or minus a 3 percent margin of error. Also, the 95 percent confidence level indicates that our survey results would be obtained in 95 out of 100 cases.

A normal distribution should be used for any populations larger than 1,000. Systematic random sampling (selecting every nth one from an alphabetical list of the population names) should be used to ensure representative survey results. At least a 50 percent survey response rate is needed to obtain the full range of opinions and minimize non-response bias. Relaxing the requirements for response rates, confidence levels, and systematic random sampling would significantly reduce the reliability of survey data—thus, degrading the integrity of the resulting improvement process—including benchmarking within or between agencies.

Agencies may need to stratify their employee, customer, and contractor populations to obtain representative samples. Stratified sampling consists of separating the elements of these populations into mutually exclusive groups (called strata) and randomly selecting samples from those strata. Stratification is especially important when it is expected that answers to survey questions may differ significantly from one stratum to another in the population (e.g., commercial firms vs. non-profit organizations, in the contractor population). It would ensure that each employee, customer, or contractor stratum is reflected according to its relative size in the population. Sampling from the overall population without stratification is more likely to result in some strata being over-represented and other strata under-represented in the survey. Without stratification, there is a risk of obtaining misleading survey responses and drawing the wrong conclusions.

For example, if an agency's contracting office expects that its contract specialists, purchasing agents, policy staff, supervisors, managers, and clerical staff would basically provide different answers to key Employee Survey questions, then it should stratify its employees by categories for sampling purposes. Also, if employee answers to survey questions are expected to differ between headquarters and field office locations, then the employees should also be broken down geographically for sampling purposes. Stratified sampling is not much more difficult to accomplish than simple random sampling. Neither survey data collection nor analyses are affected by the choice of a sampling procedure. . . .

D. Using focus groups and point-of-service questionnaires. Before bringing this chapter to a close, it would be appropriate to comment briefly on the extent to which focus groups and point-of-service questionnaires play a role in qualitative data collection. As far as point-of-service surveys are concerned (i.e., surveys done at the point where services are provided to customers), we believe that they have a legitimate place in an agency's arsenal of performance measurement tools. However, many agencies use a census to capture this type of performance information—for each and every transaction with a customer. While the information is compiled on a real-time and comprehensive basis, there's a down-side to its use: the process tends to be burdensome on the customers, and response rates tend to be lower than normal. In light of this, we recommend that agencies sample their point-of-service transactions (to reduce burden), as well as follow-up with their point-of-service survey participants (to ensure adequate response rates). Under extenuating circumstances (e.g., inability to achieve adequate response rates), it may be necessary to consider making the completion of the questionnaire a condition of the transaction. However, if the questionnaire is at all burdensome to complete, this contingency may have unintended consequences, i.e., alienation of valued customers.

With respect to focus groups, we feel that it is inherently wrong to use them as a substitute for formal survey efforts. Focus group opinions offer only anecdotal information, and are not necessarily representative of the views of the overall population of customers, employees, managers, or contractors. However, focus groups may complement or support formal survey efforts in a variety of ways. For example, agencies may use them to generate ideas for the development of survey instruments, pre-test survey instruments, implement organizational improvements downstream, etc.

DEPARTMENT OF TRANSPORTATION'S PROCUREMENT BALANCED SCORECARD

The next good example of the Balanced Scorecard in procurement is the implementation by the Department of Transportation (DOT). The material that follows has been adapted from the *Department of Transportation's Procurement Balanced Scorecard*, May 1999. The full article can be found at www.dot.gov/ost/m60/scorecard/ppmsrev.htm.

The Department of Transportation has a Procurement Performance Management System that links the GPRA requirements to procurement through a Balanced Scorecard measurement approach. Major portions of the article are included here while several key attachments are included in Appendix C.

Contents

DOT's Procurement Performance Management System Policy Principles
    Introduction
    Purpose
    Waivers
    Implementation
    Procurement Performance Management System Timeline
DOT's Procurement Performance Management System
    Introduction
    Acquisition's Strategic Path
    Procurement Performance Planning Model
DOT's Balanced Scorecard for Acquisition
    Background
    DOT'S BSC Methodology
    Key Business Drivers for Enhanced Performance
    Choosing Measurements
DOT's Three Pathways to a Balanced Scorecard
    Introduction
    The Three Pathways to DOT's Procurement BSC
    Deriving the BSC
Using Balanced Scorecard Results To Manage Performance
    Introduction
    Using BSC Results for Managed Performance
    Action Plan for Improved Performance
    Future Success
Attachments
    A—FY00 DOT-wide Procurement Performance Measurements
    B—Survey Pathway
    C—Management Information System Pathway
    D—Diagnostic Pathway
    E—Tools for Assessing Performance
    F—References and Resources

DOT'S Procurement Performance Management System Policy Principles

Introduction

This document establishes the policy principles for DOT's Procurement Performance Management System (PPMS), which links the requirements of the Government Performance and Results Act (GPRA) to procurement through the use of a Balanced Scorecard (BSC) measurement approach. DOT has chosen the BSC as its tool to gauge procurement's performance progress and to manage the risk inherent in the fiduciary responsibilities of the procurement manager. *It is also this methodology that will be used to report DOT's procurement performance under GPRA.*

The Procurement BSC contains measurements in three separate pathways, each of which connects and flows with the other. These Pathways are:

- The *Survey Pathway* uses the Performance Measurement Assessment Tool (PMAT) methodology.
- The *Management Information Systems (MIS) Pathway* uses information systems (e.g., Contract Information System) to collect data.
- The *Diagnostic Pathway* mainly uses a process and/or results-oriented assessment to evaluate performance. . . .

Purpose

The acquisition community holds a great fiduciary responsibility to the public. With the obligations of millions of dollars, we must ensure that we make wise use of public resources and act in a manner that maintains the public's trust. This includes exercising discretion, using sound business judgment, and complying with applicable laws and regulations. The purpose of this document is to set forth DOT's procurement BSC methodology, the policy principles relating to the BSC, and measurements that will flow from DOT's strategic plan to the PPMS. These measurements will gauge the performance of our fiduciary responsibility as well as gauge our progress toward our goal of becoming a world class acquisition system. The Procurement Management Council has overall responsibility for developing and maintaining the PPMS and may charter subgroups (e.g., Procurement Information Exchange Council) to help carry out this responsibility.

Procurement Performance Management System Policy Principles

- The BSC measurement approach will be the tool used to assess our performance.
- DOT wide measurements will be used.
- Operating Administration (OA) measurements (beyond the DOT wide measurements) may be used by the OA as a whole or by individual offices for their own unique needs. Data for these measures will be collected and analyzed by the OA/office utilizing the measure.
- The collection and plotting of data and submittal of the Balanced Scorecard Report to the OAs will be performed by the Senior Procurements Executive's (SPE's) office.
- An annual meeting will be held between the SPE and PMC member to discuss the OA's unique BSC results and procurement strategies. Meetings with OA field offices may be held upon request of the PMC member.
- No publication, dissemination, or comparing individual OA results will be done without prior consent of the PMC member or their representative.

OA includes the Transportation Administrative Service Center (TASC).

Waivers

Any requests for exceptions to this document shall be submitted through the HCA to the SPE. The request is to contain sufficient detail to clearly explain the basis of the request, procedures sought to be waived, and any recommended alternative action.

Implementation

This document applies to all OAs and is to be implemented by the HCA as shown in the following timeline.

Procurement Performance Management System Timeline

FY99

ACTION	TIMELINE
FY99 Budget	Completed Jun 1997
FY99 Performance Plan	Completed Sep 1997, updated Sep 1998
FY99 BSC Development	Completed Mar–Apr 1999
FY99 BSC Data Collection • Surveys • MIS	 Nov–Dec 1999 Jan 2000
FY99 Performance Report and Management Plan/Input to GPRA	Mar 2000

FY00

ACTION	TIMELINE
FY00 Budget	Completed Jun 1998
FY00 Performance Plan	Completed Sep 1998, to be updated Sep 1999
FY00 BSC Development	Jan–Mar 2000
FY00 BSC Data Collection • Surveys • MIS • Diagnostic	 Nov–Dec 2000 Jan 2001 Jan 2001*
FY00 Performance Report and Management Plan/Input to GPRA	Mar 2001

FY01

ACTION	TIMELINE
FY01 Budget	Jun 1999
FY01 Performance Plan	To be completed Sep 1999 and updated Sep 2000
FY01 BSC Development	Jan–Mar 2001
FY01 BSC Data Collection • Surveys • MIS • Diagnostic	 Nov–Dec 2001 Jan 2002 Jan 2002*
FY01 Performance Report and Management Plan/Input to GPRA	Mar 2002

*To be conducted every three years as a minimum or over the course of three years (e.g., OAs with multiple field offices).

Future timelines will follow the above FY01 timeline escalated by one year.

DOT's Procurement Performance Management System

> Coming together is a beginning.
> Keeping together is a process.
> Working together is success.
> —Henry Ford

Introduction

Uncertain times brought us face-to-face with the reality of fewer resources and less money to accomplish our mission. In 1995, to help combat these budgetary cuts, we replaced our formal Procurement Management Reviews with a less costly and less resource-intensive performance measurement system based largely on surveys provided to relevant acquisition personnel. The Performance Measurement Assessment Tool (PMAT), as this survey tool is referred, provided us with a method to assess the state of our procurement system. From the PMAT came our current use of the Balanced Scorecard (BSC) as the method by which we are deploying our strategic direction, communicating our expectations, and measuring our improvement progress. This resulted in a tool that emphasizes prevention rather than detection.

There were many statutes that impacted our choice of using the BSC to view our performance. They include: the Government Performance and Results Act (GPRA) of 1993, the Federal Acquisition Streamlining Act of 1994, the Government Management Reform Act of 1994, the Federal Acquisition Reform Act of 1995, and the Information Technology Reform Act of 1996 (the Clinger-Cohen Act). Each of these statutes, in some form, required agencies to strategically plan how they will deliver high-quality supplies and services to their customers, and specifically measure program performance in meeting their strategic commitments. DOT's strategic commitments follow many paths.

Acquisition's Strategic Path

In planning our strategic commitments, we have the opportunity through the Procurement Management Council (PMC) to look at the needs of each operating administration and consolidate the common requirements of the whole into ONE strategic objective. This is especially beneficial in the budget process where a ONE DOT approach can advance and support our budget requests. When developing our business strategies and integrating them within our planning processes, it is important that PMC members request and receive input from their field offices especially those having unique business arrangements (e.g., fee-for-service organizations). Our overall path to the BSC flows from GPRA as shown below. . . .

DOT's Strategic Path to the Balanced Scorecard
Strategic Plan—>Performance Plan—>Budget—>Performance Agreement—>
Balanced Scorecard

A synopsis of each follows:

- **DOT Strategic Plan.** The Strategic Plan is a five-year plan. It is the one document that sets forth the overall direction, vision, and mission of our agency and recognizes the requirement to set performance goals and to identify measures to gauge progress toward these goals. The acquisition portion of the Strategic Plan is under the heading "Resource and Business Process Management Strategy." . . .
- **DOT Performance Plan.** To accomplish the Strategic Plan, an annual Performance Plan is developed. This plan defines the measures, activities, and goals that, when taken together, indicate how well the agency's overall goals are being achieved. The acquisition

portion of the Performance Plan is under the heading "Resource and Business Process Management Strategy." . . .

- **Budget Process.** The budget defines the resources needed to accomplish the strategic goals. Within this process, senior acquisition managers (e.g., procurement heads) develop an acquisition budget strategy which is an integral step to strengthening budgetary requests and obtaining the resources to meet strategic planning and performance goals.
- **Performance Agreement.** A Performance Agreement is used to translate and flow down the goals and objectives of the Executive Branch through the Departments. For DOT, this top-down approach is illustrated as follows (titles may vary depending upon organizational structure):

President
⬇ Secretary of Transportation
⬇ Assistant Secretaries & Administrators of each OA
⬇ Office Directors
⬇ Office Managers/Supervisors
⬇ Employees

The goals of the Performance Plan are achieved through the efforts of DOT personnel by tasks outlined in their Performance Agreement. The achievement of these goals can be reflected in the individual's annual Performance Appraisal. By tying the appraisal to the organization's strategic goals, personnel can more fully understand the vision, mission, and goals of the organization and be rewarded for organizational accomplishments rather than just individual achievements.

Balanced scorecard-procurement performance measures. Following down the strategic planning process, more and more refined performance measures and/or tasks are utilized. These measurements are contained in [Appendix C].

The following "Procurement Performance Planning Model" illustrates how performance measures (using the BSC framework) can be developed utilizing the flow-down of the DOT strategic guidance.

Procurement Performance Planning Model

DOT Strategic Plan

Strategic Goal: Foster innovative and sound business practices as stewards of the public's resources in our quest for a fast, safe, efficient, and convenient transportation system.

DOT Performance Plan
Goal: To create a world class acquisition system.
Strategic Objectives: · Develop an acquisition workforce that meets the demands of the 21st century · Make doing business electronically our standard resulting in lower operating costs. · Improve acquisition customer satisfaction.
Measures:

Increase % of workforce meeting Clinger-Cohen educational requirements by 5% and training requirements by 50%.	Achieve a customer satisfaction rating of 85%.

Achieve a purchase card usage of 87.5% of simplified acquisition actions.	Increase use of Electronic Commerce by 5%.
Achieve Employee Satisfaction rating of 80%.	

⇩

DOT's Balanced Scorecard	

Goal: To create a world class acquisition system.

Strategic Objectives:

• To improve Customer Satisfaction.	• To make doing business electronically our standard resulting in lower operating costs.
• To improve Employee Satisfaction.	• To facilitate procurement programs that effectively apply and comply with law and regulation.
• To have business integrity, fairness, openness.	• To fulfill public policy objectives.
• To have a quality workforce meeting statutory standards.	

Measures by Perspectives:

Customer	**Employee**	**Internal Business Process (IBP)**	**and Growth**	**Finance**
–% satisfied w/ timeliness.	–% of overall employee satisfaction	–Extent IBPs facilitate program that effectively applies and complies with law and regulation	–% of employees meeting mandatory standards	–Amount of cost avoidance by using purchase cards
–% satisfied w/ quality	–% satisfied with professionalism, culture, values, empowerment	–% competitive procurement of total procurements	–Extent of reliable management information	–% of prompt pay paid vs. $ dispersed
–% satisfied w/ responsiveness, cooperation, etc. to meet mission	–% satisfied with the work environment	–% of actions using electronic commerce		–% of $ obligated for commercial items

DOT'S Balanced Scorecard for Acquisition

> Balance suggests a steadiness that results when all parts are properly adjusted to each other, when no one part or constituting force outweighs or is out of proportion to another.
> —Webster's Third New International Dictionary

Background

In 1993, the interagency Procurement Executives' Association (PEA) created the Procurement Measurement Action Team. Their task was to assess the state of the acquisition system, to identify a structured methodology to measure and improve acquisition performance, and to develop strategies for measuring the health of agency acquisition systems.

The Team found that organizations were using top-down management reviews to determine compliance with established process-oriented criteria and to certify the adequacy of the acquisition system. This method was found to lack a focus on the outcomes of the processes used and was largely ineffective in obtaining dramatic and sustained improvements in the quality of the operations.

The Team did extensive research and made site visits to leaders in performance measurement/management to identify an assessment methodology appropriate for federal organizations. The Team chose a model developed by Drs. David Norton and Robert Kaplan—the Balanced Scorecard (BSC)—because it is:

- Focused on high impact measures
- Intended to be easy and economical to use
- Balanced with emphasis on prevention rather than detection
- Customer-oriented and cross-functional
- Empowering to the procurement organization to make improvements
- Designed to compare the quality of service

The work done by this Team has formed the foundation for the BSC methodology used by DOT's acquisition community. A subsequent team was formed in 1998 by the PEA to develop a guide to a BSC. This document, "Guide to a Balanced Scorecard Performance Management Methodology," was considered a valuable resource for this document.

DOT'S BSC Methodology

DOT's BSC is a structured methodology for using performance measurement information to gauge our progress in and to help us reach our goal of creating a world class acquisition system. To achieve balance in examining the health of our organization, five overarching perspectives are used for our success. These are:

Acquisition's Five Overarching Perspectives

- Customer
- Employee
- Internal Business Processes
- Learning and Growth
- Finance

Key Business Drivers for Enhanced Performance

Within these perspectives, we focus on specific performance areas or key business drivers considered critical to DOT's acquisition function. The areas for heightened performance are:

- Cost
- Quality
- Timeliness
- Quality Work Environment
- Public Policy Fulfillment
- Integrity, Fairness, Openness
- Innovation and Streamlining
- Statutory and Regulatory Application and Compliance

These performance areas are aligned with the guiding principles of the Federal Acquisition Regulations System (Part 1) and are used by world class purchasing systems, both public and private.

Choosing Measurements

> Begin with the end in mind.
> —Stephen Covey

Once the key business drivers are chosen, it is necessary to select a method for gauging the progress toward our goal. We have selected the use of measurements as our indicators for improvement and using measurements under the five perspectives creates a balanced approach. This forms the foundation for DOT's Balanced Scorecard. (See [Appendix C] for a listing of DOT's procurement measurements.) While goals are critical to the measurement effort, a baseline normally must be developed. This may require research, experience or benchmarking with others to set the baseline necessary for determining a realistic measurement goal.

The measurements chosen are linked to DOT's Strategic Plan and focus on the outcomes necessary to meet the Plan's goals. DOT's BSC uses measurements that focus on our goal of creating a world class acquisition system. In his book, "Keeping Score," M.G. Brown provides us with some of the guidelines we consider when choosing our measurements. They include:

Measurement Guidelines

- Measures should be linked to the factors needed for success: key business drivers.
- Measures should be a mix of past, present, and future to ensure that the organization is concerned with all three perspectives.
- Measures should be based around the needs of customers, shareholders, and other key stakeholders.
- Measures should start at the top and flow down to all levels of employees in the organization. Measures need to have targets or goals established that are based on research rather than arbitrary numbers.

We also consider a number of other factors including:

- Operating administration unique needs (each OA has the opportunity to choose additional measures as needed)
- The availability and accuracy of data systems
- The impact on available resources

DOT'S Three Pathways to a Balanced Scorecard

> Even if you're on the right track, you'll be run over if you just sit there.
> —Will Rogers

Introduction

Once the key business drivers are identified and the appropriate measurements developed, it is necessary to decide how performance information will be gathered and evaluated. For DOT, the three tools used for collecting data are: surveys, management information systems, and diagnostic assessments. Each of these methods has been translated into pathways for developing and calculating measurement results. These three pathways contain the measurements, that when linked together, form DOT's Procurement Balanced Scorecard (BSC).

The Three Pathways to DOT'S Procurement BSC

The pathways to our BSC utilize the three methods we have available for collecting quantitative and/or qualitative data. Our pathways were named after these three methodologies.

- Survey Pathway (mainly Qualitative)
- Management Information System (MIS) Pathway (Quantitative)
- Diagnostic Pathway (Qualitative and/or Quantitative)

Each pathway interacts and links with the other as shown:

- The *Survey Pathway* uses the Performance Measurement Assessment Tool (PMAT) methodology.
- The *MIS Pathway* uses information systems (e.g., Contract Information System) to collect data.
- The *Diagnostic Pathway* mainly uses a process and/or results-oriented assessment to evaluate performance.

Operating administrations have significant flexibility in using the three pathways. Each, however, have core measurements from which evaluations are taken. These measurements are discussed under each path. . . .

Deriving the BSC

When the measurement results of the three pathways are linked, it provides us a full view of our progress in reaching our goal. However, before these links can be made, certain steps must be followed. These are:

- Collect the measurement data
- Compute the rating for the measurement
- Link the measurement results in graph or chart form to obtain a visual perspective

Data collection. Each of the three pathways uses a different method for collecting data.

- The *Survey Pathway*, which uses mostly qualitative data, utilizes surveys with electronic data entry capability to receive its data. The data is normally inputted by the customer, employee, and manager, and compiled by the Senior Procurement Executive's (SPE) office.
- The *MIS Pathway*, which uses quantitative data, utilizes various automated data information systems including the Contract Information System and Electronic Posting System. The data is normally inputted by the user and compiled by the SPE's office.
- The *Diagnostic Pathway*, which may use qualitative data to supplement quantitative data, mainly utilizes a manual or hands-on approach to gauge performance. Normally, the information is generated by acquisition personnel and the data compiled by independent evaluators.

Linking the measurement results. Once the data is collected and a score for each measurement is derived, the results will be displayed as a SCORECARD in chart or graph form. The charts may show results for specific measurements in the same overarching perspective, in similar functional areas, in areas having direct impacts on another, or grouped together to form a picture of the total health of the acquisition function. As much as possible, the charts will provide benchmarking data between an individual OA's measurement results and the DOT wide goal/results.

Using Balanced Scorecard Results To Manage Performance

> If there's a way to do it better . . . find it.
> —Thomas A. Edison

Introduction

We have used *performance measurement* as a method to evaluate our progress toward improving our acquisition system. *Performance management* goes a step further. It uses the results of our measurements to make positive change in the way we do business, by helping set performance goals and prioritize resources, by informing us of the need to either confirm or change current policy or program direction, and by sharing results.

For DOT, procurement performance management begins by evaluating the results of our Balanced Scorecard (BSC)—our integrated performance measurement system. *The BSC offers us the ability to consolidate, into one management document, a picture of our progress in areas needing top-level performance while also showing us if improvement in one area is causing a shortfall in another.*

Using BSC Results for Managed Performance

Role of the senior procurement executive's (SPE's) office. The SPE will, in partnership with the PMC, set DOT wide measurement goals.

The SPE's office is the point for accumulating and transferring DOT wide and OA data into a BSC chart(s) that visually depicts an OA's progress. The SPE will hold annual meetings with each PMC member (or field office representatives as requested by the PMC member) to present these DOT wide measurement results as it relates to the OA and the Department as a whole. During these meetings, management strategies for improvement will be explored which may include researching and applying the successful practices of other OAs.

The SPE's office will perform a number of outreach efforts pertaining to performance measurement. Externally, DOT will periodically participate in the benchmarking of common measurements with other Departments. When this occurs, the SPE's office will provide the results of the other Departments (along with the DOT wide results) to the OAs for internal benchmarking purposes.

Evaluating the scorecard. Understanding what a particular result really means is important in determining whether or not it has value. Collecting data by itself is not useful information, but when viewed from the context of our goals and objectives, it can be very useful. Proper analysis is imperative in determining whether or not the measurements are effective and the results are contributing to our objectives. By the use of the three pathways to the BSC—Survey, MIS, Diagnostic—we can use data to determine the level of progress we are making in reaching our goal. But how can this data be used and what do the results mean? When looking at the data results, some insight may be gained by asking the following questions:

- Does the data indicate any performance trends over time? If so, how is the trend data looking and does it reveal a shortfall in one area because of a gain in another? By comparing current and past results, we can determine if we are on the proper course.
- Were performance goals met? If not, explore what inhibited successful performance.

- Were performance goals exceeded? If so, perhaps other benefits to the organization can be gained such as operating cost reductions. Sharing such information may also spread the gain to other OAs.
- How did we compare with participating organization(s)? (Used when benchmarking.)
- Can the data be used to improve performance in areas other than the one(s) assessed or can it pinpoint specific areas for consideration? Data can help identify specific areas within the larger assessed area that need attention.
- Where should improvement efforts be focused to achieve the greatest or most needed return? Many times the amount of available resources dictates the need to focus on particular areas that will provide the most return for the resource investment.

Importance of trend data. To evaluate our performance level, trend data is perhaps the most critical of all. The more data available for a particular measurement, the better are the chances of getting an accurate picture of the progress toward our goal. While our BSC mainly uses annual data, there are many measurements, especially in the MIS Pathway, that can be reviewed on a monthly or quarterly basis. This data can provide a larger data base from which to gauge performance and to alert us to any fluctuations in performance that may need to be examined.

Key to success. The key to success is to achieve as much balance as possible for all measures on the BSC. If one measure has a deep fluctuation, care must be taken not to change too drastically to get performance back in line because it may cause problems in areas critical to a particular operation. Being able to use the measurement results to make good management decisions is the foundation of performance management. Attachment E [see Appendix C] provides a number of performance assessment tools that may be helpful when making decisions for improvement.

Action Plan for Improved Performance

Sharing results. As with any performance management system, feedback is vital for the system to grow and flourish. Retaining results without sharing them, especially among its participants, is a sure way to kill this type of system. Conversely, to share and inform, is to nurture and promote the system. Feedback can be accomplished in many ways such as through electronic mail, briefs, newsletters, and conferences. Not only is it critical to let respondents and any other interested parties know the measurement results, but it is also important to work with them to develop strategies that will be employed for improvement.

Strategies for improvement. Once measurement results are analyzed for both the DOT wide and OA measures and the areas needing improvement determined, it is time to determine the strategies needed to achieve our desired results. One of the best methods for determining the necessary strategies is to partner with your customer and/or employees. Those affected by the process are normally the best ones to reveal what needs to be done. The objective is to have the strategies lead to the goals/outcomes desired. It is those goals/outcomes that feed into the Government Performance and Results Act report.

Goal setting. Every measure needs to have an associated goal in order to know where to head, how fast to go, and when the destination is reached. Of critical importance, is to have clear, quantifiable goals for those measures contained in the Strategic and Performance Plans. When determining goals for either DOT wide or OA unique measures, the following, as required by the Government Performance and Results Act, should be considered:

- The identification of the goals in an objective, quantifiable, and measurable form;
- The operational processes, skills and technologies, and resources such as human, capital, and information needed to meet the goals;

- The basis for comparing measurement results with the desired goals; and
- The means for verifying and validating the measurement results.

Future Success

The success of our Procurement Performance Management System (PPMS) is dependent upon many factors. These include:

- Demonstrating strong support for the System at all levels of management
- Integrating procurement's critical measures into DOT's Strategic and Performance Plans
- Spreading the word as to what performance measurement and performance management is, its purpose and its benefits
- Ensuring the data (e.g., Contract Information System data) is accurate and reliable
- Promoting participation in completing surveys and other evaluation tools
- Sharing results and providing feedback to participants to help nurture and promote improvement through performance management
- Using measurement results and partnering with your customers to determine the strategies for improvement
- Translating management strategies into action for improved outcomes
- Setting goals and benchmarking results.

As we progress on our improvement journey, we expect the system to grow and become more effective. Any comments or suggestions to help lead this growth are welcome.

CHAPTER 13

The Balanced Scorecard at the National Oceanic and Atmospheric Administration

This chapter provides insight into the implementation of the BSC in three functional areas at one major organization. It shows how the National Oceanic and Atmospheric Administration (NOAA) has integrated the BSC in its systems, acquisitions, and human resources functions. The material presented is adapted from the U.S. Department of Commerce, NOAA Web site (www.rdc.noaa.gov/~itcentral/ITCproducts/ITplanning/ofacbs). This information, which was developed in October 1999, is a part of NOAA's corporate Balanced Scorecard.

SYSTEMS CORPORATE BALANCED SCORECARD

Mission
To develop and manage IT [information technology] services for NOAA & DOC [Department of Commerce]

Vision
To continue to develop a standard, cost-effective architecture

Values
To foster staff & customer relationships, planning, & opportunities to improve services and lower costs

System Map

Suppliers
- Vendors
- Contractors
- Gov't Agencies
- Management
- Staff

Customers
- OFA
- NOAA
- DOC
- Public
- Gov't Agencies

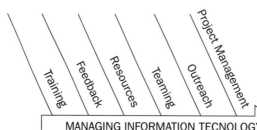

MANAGING INFORMATION TECNOLOGY

Training · Feedback · Resources · Teaming · Outreach · Project Management

Information Management · Corporate IT Security · Corporate IT Security · Tlecommunications Mgt · Operations Mgt (User Support) · Infrastructure Mgt (HW & SW) · Strategic IT Architecture P&D · Appl. Dev (ERP, programing)

Inputs
- Resources
- Policy & Regulations
- Materials
- Services
- Requirements
- Information/Knowledge

Outputs
- ADP Applications
- Strategic Plans
- Networks
- Systems
- Business Process Consulting
- IT Security
- IT Acess
- IT Support

Financial Perspective

Objectives	Performance Measure
· Decrease cost per seat for desktop applications	Cost per seat CY Cost per seat PY

Customer Perspective

Objectives	Performance Measure
· Increase % of customers reporting that expectations have been meet	# of customers reporting expectations met Total reporting

Internal Business Perspective

Objectives	Performance Measure
· Increase % of technical inquiries (TI) resolved correctly after first contact	Number of TIs resolved after first contact All inquiries

Innovation/Learning and Growth Perspective

Objectives	Performance Measure
· Increase % of skills available over skills needed by organization	Skills available Skills needed by organization

Internal Business Perspective

Objectives	Performance Measure
· Increase amount of pre-system requirements planning	· # of system requirement planning documents

ACQUISITIONS CORPORATE BALANCED SCORECARD

Mission
Fulfill client needs for supplies and services
with acquisitions that economically provide
the right deliverables on time

Vision
High customer satisfaction,
maximum use of innovation,
streamlining of processes,
optimum use of automation, compliance
with laws and regulations, unqualified audit,
CAMS implementation, trained
diversified employees

Values
Acquire high-quality supplies
and services, judiciously spend
taxpayer funds, be fair to contractors,
honesty, integrity, teamwork,
professionalism, communication

System Map

Suppliers
- Program Officials
- Contractors
- OGC
- OAM
- OFPP
- Management
- HRD, SD, FMD, FLD

Customers
- NOAA LOs
- DOC HQ
- Other DOC Bureaus
- Other Fed Agencies
- Prospective Contractors

Adequate Budget · Legal Support · Adequate IT Systems · Sufficient/Skilled Staff · Recognition · Promotions · Training

MANAGING INFORMATION TECNOLOGY

Procurement Planning · Contract Awarding · Contract Administration · Simplified Acqusition Awarding · Simplified Acqusition Admin · Purchase Card Program

Inputs
- Procurement Requests
- Planning Documents
- Offers
- Policies/Regulations
- Legal Advice
- Staff
- Budget
- IT Systems

Outputs
- Contracts/Mods
- Orders/Mods
- Interagency Agreements
- Advice
- Reports
- Purchase Card Service
- Delegations
- Training Courses
- MOUs/MOAs
- PMRs

Financial Perspective

Objectives	Performance Measure

· Administrative Cost:
  –Decrease Cost to
   Spend Ratio (CSR)
	OFA FY99 CSR
	minus OFA FY00
	CSR

Customer Perspective

Objectives	Performance Measure
· Increase % of customers reporting procured products and services delivered timely	Customers reporting timely delivery All customers surveyed
· Increase % of customers reporting satisfaction with procured products and services received	Customers reporting satisfaction All customers surveyed

Internal Business Perspective

Objectives	Performance Measure
· Decrease % of sucessful protests	Number of sucessful protests All protests
· Increase % of dollars awarded to small, minority, and women-owned businesses	Dollars awarded to small, minority, and women-owned businesses All dollars awarded

Learning and Growth Perspective

Objectives	Performance Measure
· Increase % of 1102's actively moving toward meeting mandatory OPM qualification standards	Number of 1102's demonstrating they are moving toward meeeting standards All 1102's who have not yet met standards
· Increase employee satisfaction rating of quality work environment	Index score regarding employees satisfied with work environment, measured

HUMAN RESOURCES CORPORATE BALANCED SCORECARD

Mission
Serve as a business partner in effectively managing people resources

Vision
To be a world class human resource service provider

Values
Teamwork, courtesy, service orientation, quality service, flexibility, professionalism

System Map

Suppliers
- OPM
- DOC
- NOAA/OFA & Local
- Employees
- Applicants

Customers
- NOAA & DOC Field: Managers, Supervisors, & Employees
- Job Applicants

HUMAN RESOURCE SERVICES

Work Environment
Compensation
Feedback
Leadership
Resources
Technology
Recognition Incentives
Training/Career Development

Data Input
Evaluation
Documentation
Communication
Product Development
Research
Requirement Validation

Inputs
- Customer Requests
- Laws, Regulations, & Policy
- Oversight Reviews
- Staff
- Legal Advice
- IT Hardware & Software

Outputs
- Certificates of Eligibles
- SF-50's
- Classified PD's
- Policy Issuances
- Decision Documents
- Record Maintenance
- HR Systems Support
- Info, Recommendations, & consults on: **Pay & Leave, Retirement/Benefits, RIF's, Employee & Labor Relations, Position Mgt & Classification, Recruiting/Staffing**

Existing Measures of Output

· COST	· Per Position Filled Per Employee Serviced Per Personnel Action Processed
· CYCLE TIME	· Average Time to Fill a Position (estimated)
· QUALITY	· Internal/External Evaluation Reports Number of Correction SF-50Bs
· QUANTITY	· # Clients Services # Positions Filled # SF-50Bs Processed # Separations # Promotions # Awards
· CUSTOMER SATISFACTION	· Customer Surveys

Financial Perspective

Objectives	Performance Measure
· Increase % of dollars spent for designated value-added activities (e.g., delegated examining, organizational development)	· Dollars spent divided by total dollars spent on HR minus last year figure

Customer Perspective

Objectives	Performance Measure
· Increase % of customers who report their expectations were met	· Number of customers reporting expectations met this year divided by total customers queried minus last year figure

Financial Perspective

Customer Perspective

| **Strategy**
· Determine value-add activities

· Implement DOC automation technology (e.g., COOL) upon delivery of system that meets NOAA requirements; redirect savings into value-added activities
· Utilize 17 new FTE in FY2000 | **Strategy**
· Develop and test customer service response instruments
· Refine and implement instruments

· Begin collecting baseline data |

Internal Process Perspective

| **Objectives**
· Reduce average time to issue Certificate of Eligibles

· Reduce variance in time to issue Certificate of Eligibles | **Performance Measures**
· Average number of days to issue Certs last year minus average this year divided by average number of days to issue Certs last year
· Standard deviation in number of days to issue Certs last year minus average this year divided by standard deviation number of days to issue Certs last year |

Innovation & Learning Perspective

Objectives	Performance Measures
· Increase average employee job satisfaction index score on Survey Feedback Action (SFA) · Increase average % of core competencies held by HR staff	· Average employee job satisfaction index score this survey minus the last survey divided by average of last survey · Average % of competencies held this year minus last year divided by average last year

Internal Process Perspective   **Innovation & Learning Perspective**

Strategy	Strategy
· Develop system to collect and report baseline data on number of days to issue Certificates of Eligibles · Implement DOC automated staffing system (COOL) upon delivery that meets NOAA requirements	· Use the SFA process · Determine position competencies · Assess employees' competencies · Develop IDPs

CHAPTER 14

The Balanced Scorecard in Human Resources at the Department of Energy

This chapter presents a very detailed and effective example of how the Department of Energy (DOE) developed and applied the BSC approach to the human resources (HR) function. The DOE HR Council commissioned the HR Performance Measurement Project Team to develop a systems approach to measurement. The team accomplished that objective with the aid of the Strategic Effectiveness Group, LLC and its president, John Hirsch.

On November 4, 1998, Mr. Hirsch presented a briefing on this effort. The material that follows is adapted from that briefing developed by Mr. Hirsch and Joseph Montgomery. It is presented with the approval of John Hirsch. (*Note:* Sections One and Three of the briefing are presented here; Section Two can be found in Appendix D.)

STRATEGIC MEASUREMENT SYSTEM FOR DOE CONTRACTOR HUMAN RESOURCES (SMS^{HR}): A COMPREHENSIVE APPROACH TO TAILORED STRATEGIC HR PLANNING

Introduction—A New Approach to Contractor Oversight

Through the advent of contract reform and the implementation of performance-based contracts, the Department of Energy (DOE) has determined it must redefine its oversight role in the area of Contractor Human Resources to embrace the principle of strategic management found in private industry.

The role of Human Resources (HR) in the commercial environment is evolving to the level of a strategic partner with line management in the development and accomplishment of key business goals. A central component of success for a strategic HR organization is a comprehensive, performance system which establishes goals tied to the entire organization's mission and provides feedback on the impact of and value added by HR. The SMS^{HR} is DOE's initiative to increase the effectiveness of the HR function, aligning it with both the contractor's corporate needs and those of the DOE field office and HQ.

To accomplish this objective, in 1998 the DOE HR Council commissioned the Human Resources Performance Measurement Project Team to develop a systems approach to measurement. The team established a set of criteria:

- *Activity to Result*—Emphasize the "bottom line" and results of performance, not just performance itself
- *Process to Substance*—Emphasize substantive issues, not procedural efforts unless required by statute or regulation
- *Subjectivity to Objectivity*—Emphasize objectivity while identifying strategic perspectives. HR performance measures have been traditionally "soft" which is the converse of most non-HR circumstances (e.g., Balanced Scorecard)

- *Involvement in Oversight*—Increase program oversight by de-emphasizing "daily" involvement and maintain focus on "for cause" circumstances

Additionally, in consideration of the diversity of site missions, the varying levels of HR sophistication needed, and the differences in the amount of collaboration experienced at various sites, the Project Team agreed with the RL approach that the design of any program developed should meet the following requirements:

- *Dynamic and Incremental*—Program should be phased in without an implementation "end-state"
- *Flexible and Adaptable*—Program should allow for and reflect individual circumstances of each prime contractor and measure both business management excellence and sound human resource practices
- *Collaborative*—Program should reinforce mutually developed expectations between DOE and contractor HR counterparts
- *Simplistic*—Program should be as uncomplicated as practicable
- *Accommodate*—Program should accommodate the "Balanced Scorecard" at the prime contractor level

Within the general parameters of SMS^{HR} the Project Team with the aid of the Strategic Effectiveness Group, LLC, an organizational improvement consulting team, prepared this report. The recommendations serve as a blueprint for the creation of a complex-wide process for strategic HR planning utilizing the Balanced Scorecard as its measurement oversight tool.

- Section One, "Creating an HR Balanced Scorecard," explains the logic of the process and presents the step-by-step methodology for creating a plan and the resulting scorecard.
- Section Two, "Applying the Model: Creating a BSC for a Hypothetical Hanford Contractor," is a case study that brings the process to life with examples from a variety of Hanford situations.
- Section Three, "Overview of the Balanced Scorecard," explains the purpose of the BSC and its linkage to strategic management including mission, vision, and business strategy.

Note: These three sections are prepared in a format that can be used for overhead transparency presentations.

The HR Council's expectation is that all contractor HR organizations, in collaboration with their DOE Contracting Officer, will use the process described herein to create a BSC. The process is designed to provide a product that is tailored to the particular needs of each individual operation. It is designed to focus the participants on a few key activities that will make a real difference in assisting the contractor organization in fulfilling its DOE site mission. Oversight is enhanced through specific measures that determine whether the HR function has been successful in meeting its targets. Underlying the entire process is a key assumption: the BSC is implemented in a collaborative fashion. It anticipates that interactive discussions occur throughout the process, so that the resulting BSC marries the needs of the contractor's line organization, its HR department, DOE's local program office, and contracting officer.

Section One Creating an HR Balanced Scorecard

What Are the Anticipated Requirements?
- Use of the Balanced Scorecard approach
- Contractor measures that:
- Link with contractor & DOE mission/
- Vision/strategy

- Include customer satisfaction
- Show cost and efficiency of
- Business systems
- Assess relevant aspects of
- Organizational culture
- Show compliance with laws, regulations
- A self-assessment plan (BSCA)
- A self-assessment report, based on data collected
- Participation in surveillance, validation activities by Field Office

Benefits of an HR Scorecard ("What's in It for Me?")

- Improves the HR contribution to the "bottom line"—in a visible fashion
- Gives HR a direction and strategy
- Improves the teaming relationship with DOE HR
- Makes HR look great to senior/line management
- Provides strong rationale for DOE "push backs"

Potential Concerns about the HR Scorecard ("What Is This Going To Cost Me?")

- HR will need to think strategically and in terms of contribution to the corporate mission
- Elevates DOE involvement above transactions
- Will probably require extra effort at relationship building with DOE HR
- HR will need to set priorities, disengage in some low value-added tasks

Overview: Creating an HR BSC

1) Create an HR mission, vision, strategy that are aligned with corporate and DOE Field Office HR mission, vision, strategy
2) Consider DOE, contractor drivers; identify desired organizational characteristics to support corporate, DOE HR strategies
3) Compare current status with applicable Best Practices to establish appropriate standards
4) Set performance targets for key characteristics needing change
5) Determine actions/tactics to achieve goals
6) Create measure(s) for each tactic. Specify mechanics of data collection, analysis
7) Sort measures into BSC quadrants; prioritize measures; select one or two measures for DOE oversight purposes

Preliminary Steps in BSC Preparation

Step 1

Business and Environmental Drivers

DOE Field Office		**Contractor HR Analysis:**
HR Mission	**DOE HR Tactics**	
Vision		**Based on Corporate and DOE HR Mission/Vision/Strategy, and DOE and Contractor Drivers:**
Strategy		
Corporate Mission		**1. What is Appropriate HR Mission, Vision, Strategy?**
Vision	**Corporate Tactics**	**2. What Type of Org. Does HR Need to Help Create?**
Strategy		
Collaboration between Corporate and DOE Program Office	Field Office HR Collaborates with Contractor HR Director to develop Its Tactics	**DOE HR and Corporate Review the Analysis as a Reality and Alignment Check**

RELATIONSHIPS

Understanding Field Office and Contractor HR Drivers

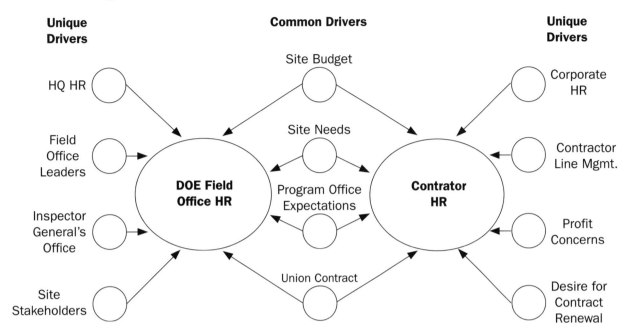

Using Desired Org. Characteristics To Drive Assessments, Goals, Tactics, and Measures

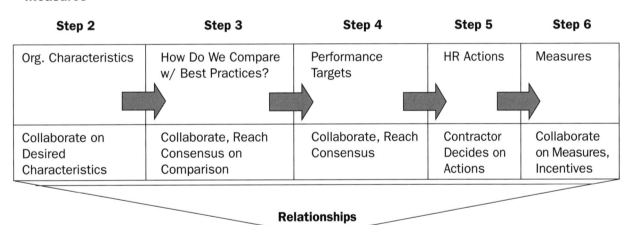

Establishing the "Mechanics"

Step 6 Continued

Measure:	How is data collected?	How often?	Who collects?

Sort Measures into a Draft BSC

Work Processes	**Culture**
Customer Satisfaction	**Finance**

Section Three Overview of the Balanced Scorecard (BSC)

Purpose of the BSC
- Indicates system-wide effectiveness, not just financial results
- Links long-term strategies with short-term actions, goals/objectives
- Builds consensus on what's important
- Communicates what's important to all levels
- Assesses degree of success of the strategy
- Builds staff alignment, accountability

Examples of Measures

Customer Satisfaction	Survey of responsiveness, quality, technical capability, overall satisfaction; number of complaints, lost customers
Culture	Survey of staff perceptions of innovation, professional dev . . . , resources; new capabilities; values, operating principles
Effective Work Processes	Cycle time, processing time, scrap/waste, output, inventory, queue time, setup time (includes white collar processes)
Financial Success	Business volume, ROI, backlog, growth in assets, capital-to-asset ratio, operating expenses

A Caution
The BSC must be built upon a sound mission, vision, and strategy. Creating a random collection of measures or using what looks good (or is popular) will not lead to success. (Kaplan & Norton, 1992, 1996)

The Strategic Management System

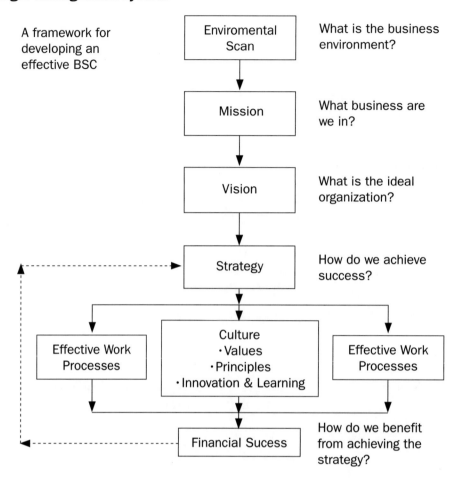

A framework for developing an effective BSC

Enviromental Scan — What is the business environment?

Mission — What business are we in?

Vision — What is the ideal organization?

Strategy — How do we achieve success?

Effective Work Processes

Culture
· Values
· Principles
· Innovation & Learning

Effective Work Processes

Financial Sucess — How do we benefit from achieving the strategy?

The Private Sector BSC

Work Processes	**Culture**
· *Innovation* · *Operations* · *Post-sale service*	· *Key values* · *Operating principles* · *Innovation* · *Learning*
Customer Satisfaction	**Finance**
· *Market share* · *Customer retention* · *Customer acquisition* · *Customer satisfaction* · *Customer profitability*	· *Revenue growth & mix* · *Cost reduction/productivity imp.* · *Asset utilization/investment strategy*
Note: bullets indicate possible topics for measure development	

Environmental Scan
- Asks customers, suppliers, stakeholders, staff, management how they view your performance
- Based on interviews, focus groups, surveys
- Requires valid, unbiased information
- Creates a clear understanding of how each group sees you
- Creates a "systems" view of the business

"Mission" Answers the Questions:
- What business are we in?
- What are we paid to provide?
- What is our value-added?
- What is our role in the organization or the market?

A sound definition of mission has *great power* to align and motivate the entire organization.

Vision
- Describes the ideal organization—one that is incredibly successful at achieving the mission
- Includes creative thinking about work processes, customers, the culture, relationships, quality, profit, professional development, etc.
- Involves a consensus of the management team, staff about the desired future

Business Strategy
- A clearly stated hypothesis about what is required for organizational success. "If we do . . . then we will succeed."
- Drives the measures used on the BSC

Strategies for Success

1) Be the leading edge innovator, technology provider, product leader
2) Be the low cost producer/supplier
3) Be the most tightly linked, integrated with the customer
4) Leverage off of unique characteristics:
   - Unique product
   - Unique, specific customers
   - Unique production characteristics
   - Unique technology
   - Unique sales approaches
   - Unique distribution features
   - Access to key natural resources

Characteristics of Sound Strategy

- Choose a single strategy—"straddling doesn't work"
- Be the best in that area
- Achieve at least minimal acceptable performance in the other three areas
- Base all actions, activities on that strategy
- Maintain flexibility—be open to opportunities

All Measures Derive from Strategy

- Finance: Are we achieving our financial objectives? Is the strategy showing bottom-line improvements?
- Customer: How is the customer reacting to our strategy? Are we providing the value-added defined by our strategy?
- Work process: Are we operating effectively, efficiently to achieve the strategy?
- Culture: Are we creating the values, skills, attitudes needed to achieve the strategy?

Chapter 15

Key Practices Driving Balanced Scorecard Outcomes

This chapter provides a unique perspective on the current state of BSC practices in the federal government. Dr. Sharon L. Caudle of the U.S. General Accounting Office (GAO), an authority in the area, developed the briefing material that follows. She has delivered this presentation at various public and the private sector seminars over the past year. The briefing material has been adapted for use here with Dr. Caudle's permission. The opinions expressed are her own and do not reflect the official position of GAO.

BALANCED SCORECARD IN GOVERNMENT 2000: KEY PRACTICES DRIVING BALANCED SCORECARD OUTCOMES

Performance-Based Government Derived from American Society for Public Administration

Policy Requirement: laws, appropriations, provisos, regulations, legislative intent
Mission: purpose, long-range goals, expected outcomes, context and structure
Program Objectives: goals, tasks, activities, benchmarks, partners, resource strategy
Product and Service Delivery: program, support, and management performance
Measure and Report: inputs, process, outputs, intermediate and final outcomes
Take Action: evaluate results and make strategy decisions
Set Mandate
Develop Mission and Goals
Set Strategies, Measures, Resources
Manage "Program" Operations
Track and Monitor
Make Strategy Decisions
Cultural and Structural Changes
Do Actual Results Match Expected Results?
Is There Accountability?
Is Strategic Adjustment Necessary?

Government Balanced Scorecard

Public Governance Responsibilities
To succeed, how should we appear as policy and resource stewards to our stakeholders?
Working Day to Day
To satisfy our clientele, how should we best work day to day in our organization and with delivery partners in extended business processes?

223

Clientele Responsibilities
To achieve our vision, how should we appear to our clientele?
Supporting Responsibilities
To achieve our responsibilities, how will we provide the right people and capabilities and technological support?

The Big Picture Questions

Meeting Public Governance Responsibilities
Meeting the Needs of Individual Clientele
Working Best Day to Day
Meeting Support Responsibilities
- What goals will meet the mission?
- What are the critical internal and external success factors?
- What measures will capture the goals in line with the agency mission and specific program purposes?
- What partners have a critical role to play?
- What means and strategies are necessary to achieve success in the short and long term?
- Who should be held accountable and when?

Public Governance Responsibilities

To succeed, how should we appear as policy and resource stewards to our stakeholders?

- Identification of stakeholders
- Key stakeholder needs and requirements
- Multiple program congruence
- Policy translation to appropriate goals with implementation accountability
- Financial and investment performance expectations
- Is the mission in line with mandates?
- Are stakeholders identified?
- Are key stakeholder needs and requirements understood and integrated?
- Are multiple/duplicate programs integrated for best policy results?
- Are mandated policies effectively translated to implementation goals?
- Are financial and investment performance restraints and expectations made clear?

Clientele Responsibilities

To achieve our vision, how should we appear to our clientele?

- Clientele requirements—customers, clients, those who are regulated
- Clientele satisfaction
- Clientele partnership, co-production
- What are the legal or regulatory policy requirements for clientele results?
- Are clientele clearly defined?
- What are clientele responsibilities in achieving results?
- Are clientele "satisfied" with program products, services, or intervention?

- Are clientele involved in defining goals, targets, measures, and strategies within legislative or regulatory parameters?

Working Day to Day

To satisfy our clientele, how should we best work day to day in our organization and with delivery partners in extended business processes?

- Delivery partner relationships
- Supplier management
- Right processes
- Operational and management process effectiveness
- Are core processes and their value chains understood and measured (time, cost, quality, quantity)?
- Is there an emphasis on comprehensive processes and interrelationships, instead of stove-piped functional tasks?
- Are there process owners to direct results and assume accountability?
- Have delivery partner/supplier roles and contributions in processes been identified—from alliances to transactional roles?

Supporting Responsibilities: Now and the Long Term

To achieve our responsibilities, how will we provide the right people and capabilities and technological support?

- Workforce competency and development
- Workforce satisfaction, retention, recognition
- Workforce size, productivity
- Access to technology and information
- Results-based climate
- Are workforce skills and competencies defined and valued?
- Is there alignment between goals and human resource systems, such as appraisals or satisfaction surveys?
- Are workforce size and productivity issues addressed?
- Is there access to information and technologies within the organization? Extended business processes?
- Does the organizational climate support achieving results, or achieving compliance?

Understanding the Linkages between Drivers and Results

Meeting the Needs of Individual Clientele
Internal/External Balanced Scorecard Key
Measures Questions
- Are the Outcomes Responsive to Public Governance and Clientele Needs?
- Do Processes Provide the Capability and Value To Meet Mission Objectives?
- Are Capabilities, Technology, and Climate Appropriate for Current and Anticipated Requirements?

Meeting Public Governance Responsibilities
Working Best Day to Day (Processes)
Meeting Support Responsibilities
Results of Past Performance
Drivers of Future Performance

Key Factors: Mission, Goals, Means, and Strategies

Internal/External Balanced Scorecard Key
Measures Question
- Are the Outcomes Responsive to Public Governance and Clientele Needs?
- Do Processes Provide the Capability and Value To Meet Mission Objectives?
- Are Capabilities, Technology, and Climate Appropriate for Current/Anticipated Requirements?
Meeting Public Governance Responsibilities
Meeting the Needs of Individual Clientele
Working Best Day to Day (Processes)
Meeting Support Responsibilities
Results of Past Performance
Drivers of Future Performance

Mission and Goals

- Mission Statement: Define current and future public purposes of the agency and programs; provide direction for goals
- Goals: Provide direction to the work, services, and activities of the organization; long-term (strategic) and shorter-period agency goals address long-term public governance and clientele (programmatic) results expectations
- Emphasis: Shift the decision-making focus from staffing and activity levels to the results of government programs—how well agency or program delivery is working
- Accountability: What results do we want
- Meeting Public Governance Responsibilities
- Meeting the Needs of Individual Clientele

Means and Strategies

Working Best Day to Day (Processes)
Meeting Support Responsibilities
- Means: Resources needed to achieve the goals—human, capital, information, and other resources
- Strategies: Processes, skills, and technologies needed to achieve the goals
- Other: Key external and contextual factors to be addressed; data resource capability
- Emphasis: Shift the decision-making focus so processes and supporting activities support the results of government programs
- Accountability: What do we think will work to achieve the outcomes we want

Coast Guard Example: From Mission to Means and Strategies

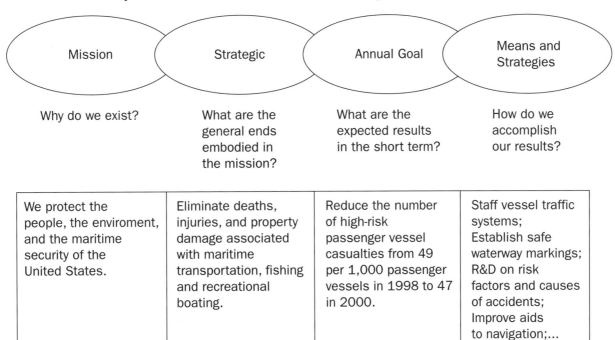

We protect the people, the enviroment, and the maritime security of the United States.	Eliminate deaths, injuries, and property damage associated with maritime transportation, fishing and recreational boating.	Reduce the number of high-risk passenger vessel casualties from 49 per 1,000 passenger vessels in 1998 to 47 in 2000.	Staff vessel traffic systems; Establish safe waterway markings; R&D on risk factors and causes of accidents; Improve aids to navigation;...

Challenges: The Government Context

- Budget misalignment with longer-term strategy and timing of performance goals
- Lack of consistency across/within administrations; policy issues drive out management
- Weak deployment systems involving other levels of government, cross-cutting program partners, and customers in "co-producing" situations
- Spotty analysis/ill-focused management attention on program "cause and effect" linkages
- Difficulty in dealing with competing policy goals and multiple stakeholders
- Difficulty in getting beyond outputs and sorting out the diverse/complex factors affecting results

The "Process" Practices—Performance-Based Management

- Top level management involved; explain the purpose, process, implementation strategies, and staff responsibilities
- Core competencies built through skill development and operational pilots
- Full management and employee participation/agreement on mission, goals, targets
- Tight mission statement and "family of plans" to implement strategies across the organization
- Target daily activities and projects to support strategies to implement goals
- Integrate goals into budgets and performance appraisals
- Construct program level collaborative relationships with clientele and program delivery partners
- Develop a data infrastructure and information systems to match goals and targets
- Use program evaluation to examine outcomes, isolate program effects from other factors, and refine the program logic model

A Logic Model: "Cause and Effect"

Workload
Other Resources
Mission and Program Purpose
External and Contextual Factors
Staff
Workload Measures: Amount of work anticipated for the program, i.e., number of clients to serve
Input Measures: Resources used to carry out the program or activity over a given time period, often used to measure process, i.e., staff and capital assets
Process Measures: Level of process activities, i.e., timeliness of activities, quality of effort, cost efficiency
Output Measures: A tabulation, calculation, or recording of activity that can be expressed in a quantitative or qualitative manner, i.e., clients served
Outcome Measures: Actual results, effectiveness, or impacts of a program or activity compared to its intended purpose, i.e., safe environment
External/Contextual Factors: Describes the broader environment that can influence inputs, outputs, and outcomes, i.e., policy, technology, or economic changes
Notes: Shows the match up between types of measures and the program logic model.

Key Practice: Establish Rationale of How a Program Delivers Results

- Build a program logic model connecting inputs to processes to outputs to outcomes
- Define complementary logic models for program delivery partners (and clientele/support functions)
- Select vital goals, targets, and measures consistent with the program logic
- Use a holistic approach to remove conflicts between goals and/or targets
- Develop a comprehensive, balanced suite of measures representing total program performance

Constructing a Program Logic Model: National Highway Traffic Safety Administration

Have New Vehicles Sold Annually with Frontal Impact Safety Information
Staff
Other Resources
Program Components
Outputs
Initial Outcomes
Intermediate Outcomes
End Outcomes
Consumers Provided with Crash-worthiness Information at Beginning of Model Year
Market Forces Motivate Car Makers To Provide Higher Levels of Occupant Protection
Greater # Vehicles on Road with High Level of Occupant Protection
Reduced Vehicle Occupant Fatalities and Injuries
Safety Performance
Workload
External and Contextual Factors
Mission and Program Purpose

Leading to Outcomes Source: James Swiss

Workload

Other Resources

Outputs are easiest to measure, being the most tangible and most immediate results. But, they are susceptible to goal displacement, i.e., what is measured can be easily increased or changed, but may not affect a link further down the chain. End outcomes are harder to measure routinely and are affected by factors outside the program.

Try to use measures where links in the chain are assumed to not break and that changes in early measures will lead to changes in outcomes.

External and Contextual Factors

Staff

Mission and Program Purpose

Notes: Shows basics of program logic model and questions [you] can ask as [you] develop.

Program Delivery Partners

Staff

Other Resources

Program Components

Outputs

Initial Outcomes

Intermediate Outcomes

End Outcomes

Workload

Staff

Other Resources

Program Components

Outputs

Initial Outcomes

Intermediate Outcomes

End Outcomes

Workload

External and Contextual Factors

Mission and Program Purpose

Accountability: Decision-Making Tiers

ENTERPRISE

Executive Information

(Mission Results)

PROGRAM

Management Information

(Program Results)

WORKPLACE/PROJECT

Activity/Task Information

(Unit Results)

Measures Align, Move from Input to Outcome

Measurement Granularity Increases from Top to Bottom

Measurement Focus and Timing

Cyclical (e.g., annual or quarterly) information that focuses on mission results; used for policy decisions and operational strategies

Periodic (e.g., quarterly or monthly) information that focuses on program results associated with management and operational improvements

Immediate (e.g., daily or weekly) information that focuses on unit or office activity and task level data used to make tactical decisions

Fitting Together (and Iterate)

Meeting Public Governance Responsibilities

Meeting the Needs of Individual Clientele

Working Best Day to Day (Processes)

Meeting Support Responsibilities

1

2

Staff

Other Resources

Program Components

Outputs

Initial Outcomes

Intermediate Outcomes

End Outcomes

Workload

External and Contextual Factors

Decision-Making Tiers

3

Mission and Program Purpose

4

Addressing Government Challenges

Meeting Public Governance Responsibilities

Meeting the Needs of Individual Clientele

Working Best Day to Day (Processes)

Meeting Support Responsibilities

Decision-Making Tiers

- Budget misalignment
- Lack of administration consistency
- Weak deployment systems with delivery partners and co-producing clientele
- Spotty analysis, problem "cause and effect" program linkages
- Dealing with competing policy goals and multiple stakeholders
- Getting beyond outputs and sorting out diverse/complex factors affecting results

CHAPTER 16

The Future of the Balanced Scorecard in the Federal Government

The Balanced Scorecard or Balanced Measures is in use at varying levels of organizations and at varying levels of effectiveness across the federal government. The breadth of use and effectiveness should only increase over time. Not the least of the impetus behind this trend will be the upcoming requirement for Senior Executive Service (SES) personnel to have their performance measured by these methods.

One of the major inhibitors to growth and effective implementation of GPRA has been the somewhat "spotty" support of top management in many federal organizations. This major change in SES performance evaluation should provide a substantial change in that area.

In many respects, the increased use of the Balanced Scorecard and Balanced Measures should be expected in the various functional areas of federal government organizations. They not only have a more precise view of what is required of them for successful operations but also are more manageable in many situations. The procurement function has been under pressure to provide faster and more effective customer service for a long time. Therefore, it is not surprising that procurement entities have gone a long way in developing the Balanced Scorecard as a measure of their success. On the other hand, trying to get large federal organizations to take on strategy and performance measurement with stakeholders, customers, and all sorts of different inputs to the process is potentially much more varied and complex.

Table 16–1 reflects the various measurement perspectives of the federal organizations discussed in this book. The first is the Kaplan/Norton[1] approach, followed by organizational perspectives and functional perspectives.

Table 16–1 Federal Government Balanced Scorecard Analysis—Measurement Perspective

Kaplan-Norton	Financial	Customer	Internal	Learning & Growth	
FAALC	Financial Stakeholder	Customer		Learning & Growth	
NUWC	Financial	Customer	Internal Business	Learning & Growth	Employee
SEO/MP		Customer	Business	Technical	People
Potential SES Guidelines	Financial Management	Customer Satisfaction	Organization Goals	Workforce	
BLM	Financial Management	Customer Satisfaction	Healthy Land	Employee Learning & Growth	
IRS	Business Results	Customer Satisfaction		Employee Satisfaction	

Report on Performance	Business	Customer	Employee		
GSA IT	Financial	Customer	Internal Business	Innovation & Learning	
DOT Proc.	Financial	Customer	Internal Business Practice	Learning & Growth	Employee
NOAA	Financial	Customer	Internal Business	Innovation/Learning & Growth	
DOE HR	Financial	Customer Satisfaction	Culture	Work Processes	
GAO BSC	Public Governance Responsibilities	Working Day to Day	Clientele Responsibilities	Supporting Responsibilities	

This book provides a wealth of information on how the concepts of the Balanced Scorecard and Balanced Measures have developed in the federal government. Now is the time to build on this foundation and develop more effective federal government organizations.

REFERENCE

1. Kaplan, Robert S., and David P. Norton. *The Balanced Scorecard.* Boston: Harvard Business School Press, 1996.

APPENDIX A

Federal Aviation Administration Logistics Center, Oklahoma City

The following material is adapted from the Federal Aviation Administration Logistics Center, *Strategic Planning, Vision of the Future,* August 1992.

CURRENT BUSINESS MODEL

Based on the Environmental Assessment following is a description of our Current Business Model:

KEY ELEMENT

DESCRIPTION

NAS LOGISTICS SUPPORT IN FAA: DECENTRALIZED
AXX-50'S, ALM~AMQ, AVN, ASU,
AND FAALC

FAALC MISSION:

CUSTOMERS:

LINES OF BUSINESS:

RESOURCES:

PEOPLE:

ORGANIZATION:

DEPOT LEVEL SUPPLY SUPPORT-EQUIPMENT FOCUS

AAF, AVN, MMAC, AXA, OTHER GOVERNMENT AGENCIES, INTERNATIONAL

PRODUCT ORIENTED, INVENTORY, REPAIR, DISTRIBUTION, ACQUISITION, WAREHOUSING, DEPOT LEVEL LOGISTICS INFORMATION SERVICES

FUNDING (F&E, OPS, R&D) BASED ON FRAGMENTED BUDGET PROCESS. FAALC RESOURCES/REQUIREMENTS BASED ON COMMISSIONINGS AND DEMAND.

SPECIALIZED/FUNCTIONAL SKILLS

FUNCTIONAL ALIGNMENT-"STOVEPIPE"

ENVIRONMENTAL ASSESSMENT CONCLUSIONS—So what does all this mean?

Having assessed the environment today, and the environment tomorrow, and constructed the current business model, what would be the result if we continued to do business in the same manner as we do today in the environment of tomorrow?

Well, we would not have as much workload, we would not be a key player in the management of NAS logistics support, and we would not be very efficient. It is unlikely the FAA or anyone else would ask us to provide any services, and our mission would be diminished. In short we might cease to exist, or at least be a very small operation.

BUT ALL IS NOT LOST! *We have time to influence the changes being made, and shape our own Future.* In the next section you will see how each of the key elements of our current business model must change if we are to continue to perform our mission in the 21st century.

PART 4
FAALC FUTURE BUSINESS MODEL

Based on the information gathered and analyzed in the Environmental Assessment the FAALC Management Team developed the following vision for the FAALC.

THE FAALC VISION FOR THE FUTURE

The FAA Logistics Center is the preferred choice for logistics support of the National Airspace System (NAS).

After reviewing all the information gathered in the Environmental Assessment the FAALC Management Team was faced with a decision . . . What do we want to be in the future? The above statement is the overriding vision which provided the focus for development of the future business model and the major strategies to close the gaps between today and tomorrow. All strategies, objectives, and decisions made in the strategic planning process will support this vision.

FUTURE BUSINESS MODEL

Based on analysis of the potential changes brought about by the external factors discussed in the preceding Environmental Assessment, the FAALC Management Team developed the following future business model. This model reflects what the Management Team feels we must look like in order to achieve our vision and continue to play a leading role in the FAA Logistics Support process.

- NAS LOGISTICS SUPPORT IN FAA: INTEGRATED—LIFE CYCLE MANAGEMENT
- FAALC MISSION: SYSTEMS FOCUSED—LIFE CYCLE
                                                          MANAGEMENT SUPPORT

- CUSTOMERS: AF, AT AVN, MMAC, AXA, OTHER GOV'T
                             AGENCIES INTERNATIONAL *(CONTRACTORS?)*

- LINES OF BUSINESS: CONTRACT MANAGEMENT, *NATIONAL*
                             INFORMATION SERVICES, CENTRALIZED FIELD
                             MAINTENANCE, ENHANCED DEPOT LEVEL
                             SERVICES, INVENTORY MANAGEMENT,
                             DISTRIBUTIVE OPERATIONS

- RESOURCES: FAA FUNDING BASED ON FAA LIFE CYCLE
                             MANAGEMENT BUDGETING PROCESS. FAALC
                             RESOURCES AND REQUIREMENTS BASED ON
                             OUR ABILITY TO SELL OR PRODUCE PRODUCTS
                             OR SERVICES.

- PEOPLE: MULTI-SKILLED, PRODUCT TEAM FOCUS

- ORGANIZATION: PRODUCT/SERVICE BASED, FEWER LAYERS,
                             TEAM CONCEPT

PART 5
GAP ANALYSIS

During this step the Management Team compared the Current Business Model to the Future Business Model and determined what are the obstacles we must overcome to close the gaps. The key elements of the current and future business model, i.e., NAS Logistics Support in FAA, FAALC Mission, Customers, Lines of Business, Resources, People, and Organization, are the key issue areas to be addressed as we develop strategies to close the gaps.

Even a quick comparison of the Current Business Model and the Future Business Model reveals some pretty obvious differences between today and the future. However, there are some important issues associated with each gap that represent obstacles to reaching the desired outcome. These are strategic issues. To be included as a strategic issue the FAALC must be able to solve the problem. Normally strategic issues concern how the FAALC (internal) relates to the environment it operates within (external). . . .

PART 6
STRATEGY DEVELOPMENT

At this point the Management Team must answer the question, "How do we address the strategic issues associated with each gap?" The answers to these questions are the basic strategies necessary to reach the desired outcome. A *summary* of the Gaps, Strategic Issues, and some of the specific strategies developed to date by the Management Team follows this section.

As the Management Team delved into the strategy development phase a prominent theme began to develop. Each of the specific strategies developed fell into one of the four following broad strategies:

Streamline/enhance current operations
Increase competitiveness
Enter new lines of business
Implement a new way of doing business—Life Cycle Management

The Management Team considers these four "broad" strategies the **foundation** of our strategic plan. The Management Team is committed to these basic strategies and believes firmly these strategies will assure the FAALC is a vital part of the FAA in Oklahoma for years to come.

The specific strategies discussed and proposed by the Management Team are listed in the next section, however, these are just a starting point and open for comment by any FAALC employee. Collectively, we, all employees of the FAALC, hold the future of the FAALC. The Management Team has tried to provide a basic design for the future. Now we all need to work together to build the bridge to tomorrow.

PART 7
GAP AND STRATEGY SUMMARY

The gaps, issues, and strategies are discussed by key issue area:

NAS LOGISTICS SUPPORT IN FAA
FAALC MISSION
CUSTOMERS
LINES OF BUSINESS
RESOURCES (FINANCIAL)
PEOPLE
ORGANIZATION

KEY ISSUE AREA: NAS LOGISTICS SUPPORT IN FAA

GAP:

Lack of integration between various organizations within FAA which have logistics support responsibilities.

DESIRED OUTCOME:

The FAALC uses an automated national life cycle management planning process. The FAALC performs integrated planning in support of NAS logistic support and provides the appropriate information to the national information system. FAALC planning processes consider the needs of the customer and user.

STRATEGIC ISSUES:

FAALC role in the Integrated Product Development System. Capability to compile complete and accurate supportability requirements. NAILS implementation. Sparing Model.

STRATEGIES:

Define FAALC role in Integrated Product Development System process. Develop plan of action to assure FAALC role is officially recognized by other FAA organizations.

Develop plan to achieve integrated automation technology, system design, acquisition processes, and logistics support analysis through adherence to the CALS initiative.

SPONSOR: AML-200

KEY ISSUE AREA: FAALC MISSION

GAP:

Mission expanded beyond current Depot Level Supply Support and Maintenance to Life Cycle Management Support.

DESIRED OUTCOME:

The FAA Logistics Center is the preferred choice throughout the FAA and non-FAA organizations for logistics support. The FAALC influences NAS system design and maintenance *planning* integration to ensure logistics supportability over the systems life cycle. Through highly integrated automation, the FAALC is the expert on contract management and distributive operations. The FAALC is in partnership with our customers for life cycle management and cost accountability.

The FAALC Mission in the future drives the development of all other gaps and strategies described in this plan. Execution of the strategies and action plans developed in the other key issue areas will close this gap. Therefore, strategic issues and strategies are not described for this gap.

KEY ISSUE AREA: CUSTOMERS

GAP: Lack of strong customer partnerships.

DESIRED OUTCOME:

The FAALC, in partnership with the FAA's life cycle managers and field maintenance activities, share[s] accountability for all aspects of NAS system planning and logistics support. Through automated supply support and feedback systems, customers actively participate with the FAALC in integrated logistics support planning budget formulation/execution, inventory management, and spares control. Continuous customer participation along with feedback enhances the efficiency and economy of the NAS.

STRATEGIC ISSUES:

Customers are also sometimes our competitors—protection of turf may be barrier to development of partnerships. Inadequate customer feedback mechanisms and processes. Customer perception of FAALC.

STRATEGY:

Develop plan to build customer partnerships and break down organizational barriers. Enhance customer feedback system, develop automated system to provide information which is tracked, queued, and responded to on-line/real time. Compile information on all current FAALC customer feedback mechanisms, identify gaps in information, and develop process for assimilating feedback to provide meaningful management information.

SPONSOR: AML-500

KEY ISSUE AREA: LINES OF BUSINESS

GAP:

There are four major gaps associated with this key issue area:
(1) Contract Management
(2) Centralized Field Maintenance
(3) National Logistics Information Services
(4) Configuration Management

GAP (1) Contract Management.

Lines of business do not include contract management responsibility for Airway Facilities logistics support and maintenance contracts.

DESIRED OUTCOME:

The FAALC is responsible for managing the FAA's NAS logistics support and system maintenance contracts.

STRATEGIC ISSUES:

Gaining support from HQ, and customers for transfer of function to FAALC.
Developing contract management skills.
Transfer of authorizations.
Improving program to assure we obtain best value for the FAA.
Overlap with AOS.
Interface with AMQ and ASU.
Budget transfer.
Issue authority.
Contractor performance evaluation.
Contracting process weakness, e.g., excessive lead time, inadequate statements of work/
   requirements, etc.

STRATEGIES:

Develop plan for FAALC to assume CMLS contract management functions currently performed by ALM.
Develop plan to assure contractors provide quality products that meet ISO 9000 requirements.
Study local contracting process to assure most effective lead time for all FAALC customer requirements.

SPONSOR: AML-600

APPENDIX B

Veterans Benefits Administration Systematic Technical Accuracy Review (Star) Checklist—Rating

The following material is adapted from the Veterans Benefits Administration, Department of Veterans Affairs, *Systematic Technical Accuracy Review Program for Compensation and Pension Claims Processing*, November 24, 1998, Circular 21-98-3.

STAR CHECKLIST—RATING

	YES	NO	N/A
Well Grounded Claim			
A1) Was concept of "Well Grounded Claim" properly addressed?			
Address All Issues			
B1) Were all claimed issues addressed?			
B2) Were all inferred issues addressed?			
B3) Were all ancillary issues addressed?			
Proper Development			
C1) If the claim is well grounded, does the record show a documented attempt to obtain all indicated evidence (including a VA exam, if required) prior to deciding the claim? *IF NO, SPECIFY DEFICIENCY:* ____ Private Medical ____VAMC Records ____Service Records ____VA Exam ____Medical Opinion ____Other			
C2) If a VA examination was requested, was that examination necessary and if an opinion was requested was the opinion an appropriate medical (not legal) question?			
C3) If the claim was well grounded, was evidence received prior to denying the claim? If not, is there documentation to show that the claimant was given an opportunity to obtain and submit the evidence? *IF NO, SPECIFY DEFICIENCY:* ____Private Medical ____VAMC Records ____Service Records ____VA Exam ____Evidence of Continuity ____Evidence of Presumptive SC			
Grant or Deny			
D1) Was the grant or denial of all issues correct?			
D2) Was the percentage evaluation assigned correct?			
D3) Was the combined evaluation correct?			

	YES	NO	N/A
Award Actions			
E1) Are all effective dates affecting payment correct?			
E2) Were payment rates correct?			
Reasons & Bases			
F1) Was all applicable evidence discussed?			
F2) Was the basis of each decision explained?			
Notification			
G1) Was notification sent?			
G2) Was the Power of Attorney indicated and correct?			
G3) Was the notification correct?			
G4) Were appeal rights included?			
Administrative			
H1) List total number of Rating Issues.			
H2) List number of Rating Issues done incorrectly.			
H3) Special Issue Case? ____POW ____Radiation ____GW ____Agent Orange ____PTSD ____BVA Remand			

FOR EACH "NO" ANSWER RECORDED, PROVIDE A *BRIEF* NARRATIVE SUMMARY OF THE ERROR AND STATUTORY, REGULATORY, JUDICIAL, OR MANUAL REFERENCES ON THE ATTACHED NARRATIVE SUMMARY SHEET.

Systematic Technical Accuracy Review
Compensation & Pension Service
Narrative Summary of Error(s)

End Product _____   Claim Number _____

Benefit Type _____   Name _____

NARRATIVE SUMMARY OF EACH ERROR ("NO" ANSWER ON FRONT PAGE) AND STATUTORY, REGULATORY, JUDICIAL, OR MANUAL REFERENCE

REMARKS

DATE   SIGNATURE OF REVIEWER   REVIEWER LOCATION

ACTION TAKEN BY REGIONAL OFFICE

DATE   SIGNATURE   TITLE

INSTRUCTIONS AND GUIDELINES—RATING REVIEW

These instructions and guidelines have been developed to promote consistency and uniformity in the review of cases selected for the Systematic Technical Accuracy Review (STAR) program. Use these instructions/guidelines in conjunction with the STAR Checklist—Rating.

For the purpose of measuring technical accuracy under the STAR program, a case is considered either "accurate" or "in error." A case will be considered "accurate" when all of the questions for each of seven elements indicated on the STAR Checklist—Rating are answered "YES" or "N/A." The seven elements are: A) Well Grounded Claim, B) Address All Issues, C) Proper Development, D) Grant or Denial, E) Effective Dates, F) Reasons and Bases, and G) Notification. A case will be considered "in error" if the answer to any question for any element is "NO."

For each case reviewed, a STAR Checklist must be completed and all 18 questions answered. A "YES" response indicates that the activity associated with the question was completed accurately. A "NO" response indicates that the activity associated with the question was "in error." Indicate "N/A" if the question is not applicable to the case under review, or if a "NO" response was previously recorded for the only issue subject to review. A narrative summary is required with statutory, regulatory, judicial, or manual references for any "error" or "NO" answer recorded.

A "NO" response will be recorded only if an action/decision is clearly in error. An error includes failure to allow benefits based upon application of the doctrine of reasonable doubt when a case is in equipoise (38 CFR 3.102). A judgment variance such as "difference of opinion" or "better rating practice" will not be considered an error but may be noted as a remark or comment.

Improper application of not well grounded claim will be considered an error. If a claim is found to be not well grounded, failure to meet the duty to inform requirement (that is to indicate evidence necessary to well ground a claim) constitutes an error.

If upon folder review there is no documented action to warrant an end product credit, or an incorrect end product was taken, that fact should be recorded in the heading area of the checklist and the checklist should not be otherwise completed. (Any apparent problems identified may be noted as a remark or comment.) The third digit modifier will not be considered for purposes of establishing whether or not an end product subject to review is considered correct.

WELL GROUNDED A) Was "well grounded" concept properly addressed?	Was the claim properly determined to be "well grounded" before applying duty to assist? If the claim was denied as "not well grounded" was that a correct decision? Was claimant informed of evidence required to "well ground" his/her claim (duty to inform)?
ADDRESS ALL ISSUES	The STAR Rating review is, generally, focused on end products associated with original and reopened claims and appellate issues. Other issues such as dependency, income, net worth, withholdings/ recoupments, incompetency, etc., when applicable to a case selected under STAR, will be reviewed as part of that end product.

B1) Were all claimed issues addressed?	A "claimed issue" is any benefit specifically mentioned by the applicant or his/her representative. Since a claim may be received through any means of communication, each document in the file must be checked to ensure that all issues have been addressed.
B2) Were all inferred issues addressed?	An "inferred issue" is not defined by regulation. An "inferred issue" is often derived from the consideration or outcome of a "claimed issue." COVA has stated that "An issue may not be ignored or rejected merely because the veteran did not expressly raise the appropriate legal provision for the benefit sought." A list of some, but not all, "inferred issues" is included in M21-1, Part VI, Chapter 3. Not included in this list, but also considered to be "inferred" are unclaimed chronic diseases or injuries with residuals which are identified during review of the SMRs and identified unclaimed compensable presumptive diseases within the time period allowed by statute.
B3) Were all ancillary issues addressed?	"Ancillary issues" are enumerated in M21-1, Part VI, Chapter 4.
PROPER DEVELOPMENT	
C1) If the claim was well grounded, does the record show a documented attempt to obtain all indicated evidence (including VA exam, if required) prior to denial of the claim?	All indicated development must be completed before deciding a claim, unless allowance is warranted based on the evidence of record. (Refer to the *Summary of Significant Holdings of the United States Court of Veterans Appeals*, Third Edition, issued by the C&P Service in February 1996 for a good discussion of VA's duty to assist.)
C2) If a VA examination was requested, was that examination necessary and if an opinion was requested was the opinion an appropriate medical (not legal) question?	If a VA examination was requested was that examination necessary and appropriate? Was there already sufficient medical evidence of record to rate the claim? (See 38 CFR 3.326 [b]&[c].) While requesting an examination is generally a judgment area with considerable latitude, that judgment must be exercised within a reasonable range. To be called an error, the record must contain evidence that is clearly and unmistakably sufficient for adjudication of the claim. Instances where the evidence is not irrefutably sufficient, but where the evidence would be considered adequate by most reviewers will simply be recorded as a comment. Requests for medical opinions on legal issues such as "is a condition service connected" constitute error.
C3) If the claim was well grounded, was all evidence received prior to denying the claim? If not, is there documentation to show the claimant was given an opportunity to obtain and submit the evidence?	An exam is required in a claim for increased evaluation for a service-connected disability when the claimant cites increased symptoms, unless medical evidence is received which is sufficient to evaluate the claimed increase. Also, an exam is required when SMRs or other medical evidence is too old to evaluate an issue. It is anticipated that

	judgment calls made by regional office personnel on the need for examinations will, at times, differ from those of the reviewer. These differences of a judgmental nature will not be considered errors, but should be noted in REMARKS.
GRANT OR DENY	
D1) Was the grant or denial of all issues correct?	If a VA examination report was the basis for a rating decision, was that report adequate and sufficient for rating purposes? Does the evidence of record support the decision according to applicable law and regulation?
	If applicable to the case being reviewed, issues such as dependency, income, withholdings and recoupments, hospitalization, etc., must be considered when deciding whether the payment rates are correct.
	Any error called in this element must be the equivalent of a clear and unmistakable error. An error includes failure to allow benefits based upon application of the doctrine of reasonable doubt when a case is in equipoise (38 CFR 3.102). A judgment variance such as "difference of opinion" or "better rating practice" should be noted in REMARKS but will not be considered an error.
	Deficiencies invisible to the claimant such as award reason codes or entitlement codes should not be called. Such deficiencies should be noted in the REMARKS section of the form.
D2) Was the percentage evaluation assigned correct?	A judgment variance with regard to percentage of evaluation will not be considered an error but should be noted in REMARKS. The only possible judgment variance is when the evidence of symptomatology is divided between two evaluation criteria and the disability picture is not clear enough to conclusively apply 38 CFR 4.7.
D3) Was the combined evaluation correct?	Question D3 is self-explanatory.
AWARD ACTIONS	
E1) Are all effective dates *affecting payment* correct?	Question E1 is self-explanatory.
E2) Were payment rates correct?	Question E2 is self-explanatory.
REASONS AND BASES	Simply summarizing evidence and stating a conclusion does not constitute "reasons and bases." In *Gabrielson v. Brown*, 7 Vet. App 36 (1994), the court stated: " . . . fulfillment of the reasons and bases mandate requires the decision maker to set forth the precise basis for its decision, to analyze the credibility and probative value of all material evidence submitted by and on behalf of a claimant in support of the claim, and to provide a statement

	of its reasons and bases for rejecting any such evidence." Failure to do this on an issue is an error.
F1) Was all applicable evidence discussed?	Question F1 is self-explanatory.
F2) Was the basis of each decision explained?	Question F2 is self-explanatory.
NOTIFICATION	This element includes Predetermination and Contemporaneous Notification, when applicable (38 CFR 3.103).
G1) Was Notification sent?	Question G1 is self-explanatory.
G2) Was the Power of Attorney indicated and correct?	Question G2 is self-explanatory.
G3) Was the notification correct?	It is essential that correspondence to claimants be viewed, to the extent possible, from the claimant's perspective. Notification must: –Be factually correct, –Address all issues, –Be as direct and concise as possible, –Be logically laid out so thought sequences are not broken, and –Be free from apparent contradictory statements.
G4) Were appeal rights included?	Question G4 is self-explanatory.

Regional Office Number _____

End Product _____

End Product Correct? _____Yes ____No

Claim Number _____

Name _____

STAR CHECKLIST—AUTHORIZATION

	YES	NO	N/A
Well Grounded Claim			
A) Was concept of "Well Grounded Claim" properly addressed?			
Address All Issues			
B1) Were all claimed issues addressed?			
B2) Were all inferred issues addressed?			
Proper Development			
C1) If the claim is well grounded, does the record show a documented attempt to obtain all indicated evidence prior to deciding the claim?			
C2) Was all necessary evidence received prior to deciding the claim; if not, was the claimant properly advised of the evidence requirements before the decision was made and of his/her responsibilities in that regard?			
Income Issues			
D1) Was Net Worth determination correct?			
D2) Was income counted in the correct reporting period?			
D3) Was total family income counted properly?			
D4) Were all deductions including unreimbursed medical expenses calculated correctly ?			
Dependency Issues			
E1) Was a dependent spouse correctly established?			
E2) Were dependent children correctly established?			
E3) Were dependent parents correctly established?			
E4) Was a surviving spouse correctly established?			
E5) Were surviving children correctly established?			
E6) Were SSNs on record for all dependents?			
E7) Were required formal apportionment decisions completed and correct?			
Burial Issues			
F1) Was the proper claimant paid?			
F2) Were transportation charges applied correctly?			
F3) Was the Burial/Plot/Headstone payment correct?			
Accrued Benefits Issues			
G1) Was the proper claimant paid?			
G2) Was the correct amount paid?			
Hospital Adjustments			
H1) Was the reduction, or suspension, correct?			
H2) Was restoration of benefits correct?			
Due Process Issues			
I1) Was a predetermination notice sent?			
I2) Was the notice fully informative?			
I3) Was the claimant given 60 days before the due process period expired?			

	YES	NO	N/A
Effective Dates			
J) Are all payment dates correct?			
Denials			
K1) Was all applicable evidence discussed?			
K2) Was the basis of each decision explained?			
Notification			
L1) Was notification sent?			
L2) Was the Power of Attorney indicated and correct?			
L3) Was the notification correct?			
L4) Were appeal rights included?			

FOR EACH "NO" ANSWER RECORDED, PROVIDE A *BRIEF* NARRATIVE SUMMARY OF THE ERROR AND STATUTORY, REGULATORY, JUDICIAL, OR MANUAL REFERENCES ON THE REVERSE OF ATTACHED NARRATIVE SUMMARY SHEET.

Systematic Technical Accuracy Review
Compensation & Pension Service
Narrative Summary of Error(s)

End Product _____ Claim Number _____

Benefit Type _____ Name _____

NARRATIVE SUMMARY OF EACH ERROR ("NO" ANSWER ON FRONT PAGE) AND STATUTORY, REGULATORY, JUDICIAL, OR MANUAL REFERENCE

REMARKS

DATE   SIGNATURE OF REVIEWER   REVIEWER LOCATION

ACTION TAKEN BY REGIONAL OFFICE

DATE   SIGNATURE   TITLE

INSTRUCTIONS AND GUIDELINES—AUTHORIZATION REVIEW

These instructions and guidelines have been developed to promote consistency and uniformity in the review of cases selected for the Systematic Technical Accuracy Review (STAR) program. Use these instructions/guidelines in conjunction with the STAR Checklist—Authorization.

For the purpose of measuring technical accuracy under the STAR program, a case is considered either "accurate" or "in error." A case will be considered "accurate" when all of the questions for each of twelve elements indicated on the STAR Checklist—Authorization are answered "YES" or "NA." The twelve elements are: A) Well Grounded Claim, B) Address All Issues, C) Proper Development, D) Income Issues, E) Dependency Issues, F) Burial Benefits, G) Accrued Benefits Issues, H) Hospital Adjustments, I) Due Process Issues, J) Effective Dates, K) Denials, and L) Notifications. A case will be considered "in error" if the answer to any question for any element is "NO."

For each case reviewed, a STAR Checklist must be completed and all 33 questions answered. A "YES" response indicates that the activity associated with the question was completed accurately. A "NO" response indicates that the activity associated with the question was "in error." Indicate "N/A" if the question is not applicable to the case under review or if a "NO" response was previously recorded for the only issue subject to review. A narrative summary is required with statutory, regulatory, judicial, or manual references for any "error" or "NO" answer recorded.

A "NO" response will be recorded only if an action/decision is clearly in error. An error includes failure to allow benefits based upon application of the doctrine of reasonable doubt when a case is in equipoise (38 CFR 3.102). A judgment variance such as "difference of opinion" will not be considered an error but should be noted in REMARKS on the reverse side of the form.

If upon folder review there is no documented action to warrant an end product credit, or an incorrect end product was taken, that fact should be recorded in the heading area of the checklist and the checklist should not be otherwise completed. (Any apparent problems identified may be noted as a remark or comment.) The third digit modifier will not be considered for purposes of establishing whether or not an end product subject to review is considered correct.

WELL GROUNDED	
A) Was concept of well grounded claim properly addressed?	While for most authorization issues "not well grounded" will generally not be an issue, for those cases where "well grounded" may be a factor, was the concept of "well grounded" properly applied before applying duty to assist? If the claim was denied as "not well grounded" was that a correct decision? Was the claimant informed of evidence required to "well ground" his/her claim (duty to inform)?
ADDRESS ALL ISSUES	While, generally, authorization issues are more limited in scope than rating issues, the reviewer must ensure that all issues associated with the claim under review have been considered.
B1) Were all claimed issues addressed?	A "claimed issue" is any benefit specifically mentioned by the applicant or his/her representative. Since a claim may be received through any means

	of communication, each document in the file must be checked to ensure that all issues have been addressed.
B2) Were all inferred issues addressed?	An "inferred issue" is not defined by regulation. An "inferred issue" is often derived from the consideration or outcome of a "claimed issue." COVA has stated that "An issue may not be ignored or rejected merely because the veteran did not expressly raise the appropriate legal provision for the benefit sought."
PROPER DEVELOPMENT	
C1) If the claim is well grounded, does the record show a documented attempt to obtain all indicated evidence prior to denial of the claim?	All indicated development must be completed before deciding a claim unless allowance is warranted based on the evidence of record. (Refer to the *Summary of Significant Holdings of the United States Court of Veterans Appeals*, Third Edition, issued by the C&P Service in February 1996 for a good discussion of VA's duty to assist.)
C2) If the claim was well grounded, was all evidence received prior to deciding the claim? If not, is there documented follow-up to show that the claimant was given the opportunity to obtain and submit the evidence?	Once VA's duty to assist has been triggered by submission of a well grounded claim, all indicated development must be accomplished. The duty to assist ends when all relevant evidence is obtained, or cannot be obtained despite reasonable efforts, or benefits are granted. While allowances must be substantiated, there is no duty to assist requirement to develop additional records when entitlement can be established on the evidence of record. VA's efforts to assist where the evidence requested has not been received must be documented in any adverse decision.
INCOME ISSUES	
D1) Was Net Worth determination correct?	Net worth is a factor in determining eligibility for Section 306 pension, Improved Pension, and dependency of parents.
D2) Was income counted in the correct reporting period?	IVAP is determined on a calendar year basis for Section 306, old law pension, and parents' DIC. IVAP for Improved Pension is, generally, "annualized" from the date of receipt. Monthly income is determinative to establish dependency of parents
D3) Was total family income counted properly?	Income of family members can affect the monthly benefit rate. The number of family members can affect the maximum allowable income limit.
D4) Were all deductions including unreimbursed medical expenses calculated correctly?	Unique exclusions apply to each benefit type. Rules are contained in 38 CFR 3.250 through 3.277. Exclusions/deductions from income are unique to each benefit. Rules are contained in 38 CFR 3.261, 3.262, and 3.272.
DEPENDENCY ISSUES	Establishment of qualifying dependents can affect the benefit rate payable. Two issues must be resolved: relationship and dependency. Dependency may be assumed or may require development.

	Dependency is secondary to the primary resolution of relationship.
E1) Was a dependent spouse correctly established?	38 CFR 3.50 is the basic rule. Further definitions and development requirements are contained in 38 CFR 3.50 through 3.60 and 3.200 through 3.216. The scope of this and other dependency questions includes preparation of a justifiable Administrative Decision when required.
E2) Were dependent children correctly established?	The issues of date of birth, relationship, and, in some cases, custody must be properly resolved. Development for school attendance may be required.
E3) Were dependent parents correctly established?	38 CFR 3.59 is the basic rule. Relationship and dependency must be properly established.
E4) Was a surviving spouse correctly established?	38 CFR 3.50 (b) is the basic rule.
E5) Were surviving children correctly established?	38 CFR 3.57 is the basic rule.
E6) Were SSNs on record for all dependents?	Development for SSNs is mandatory under 38 CFR 3.216.
E7) Were required formal apportionment decisions completed and correct?	The basic rules are contained in 38 CFR 3.450 through 3.461.
Burial Benefits	Included in this element are the full range of both service-connected and nonservice-connected burial benefits. The basic rules are contained in 38 CFR 3.1600 through 3.1612. Development should not create an unnecessary burden on the veteran's survivors. Beginning with this element, questions are phrased in terms of payment. Denials are equally applicable.
F1) Was the proper claimant paid?	In addition to the obvious wording of this question, a "NO" response is warranted if the proper claimant was not identified or the proper claimant was erroneously denied payment.
F2) Were transportation charges applied correctly?	38 CFR 3.1606 is the basic rule.
F3) Was the Burial/Plot/Headstone payment correct?	The basic rules are contained in 38 CFR 3.1600 through 3.1612.
Accrued Benefits Issues	The basic rules are contained in 38 CFR 3.1000 through 3.1009. Again, denials are equally applicable.
G1) Was the proper claimant paid?	Payment may be based on relationship or made as reimbursement.
G2) Was the correct amount paid?	Payment as reimbursement requires development of expense items. Payment based on relationship requires application of specific time limits.
Hospital Adjustments	The basic rules are contained in 38 CFR 3.551 through 3.559. Timely exchange of information between VA medical facilities and regional offices is crucial in order to minimize overpayments.

H1) Were required reductions accomplished?	The benefit payable and type of VA care are critical for proper application of these rules. The existence of dependents can affect the necessity for reduction or suspension.
H2) Was the reduction, suspension, or temporary increase correct?	See above.
H3) Was restoration of benefits correct?	The type of benefit and medical discharge can affect restoration.
Due Process Issues	The basic rule concerning notice is found at 38 CFR 3.103. Within that regulation, at 3.103 (b) (2), are provisions for due process associated with adverse actions. Additional instructions for implementation are found in M21-1, PT. IV, Chapter 9. Strict adherence to these procedures is necessary both from the customer's perspective and the government's.
I1) Was a predetermination notice sent?	This notice is based upon a proposed, rather than final, action. Contemporaneous notice and no notice situations are not included.
I2) Was the notice fully informative?	*All* of the elements specified in M21-1, PT. IV, 9.03 must be included in this notice.
I3) Was the claimant given 60 days before the due process period expired?	Control is maintained under end product 600. A 60 day waiting period is required unless the claimant agrees to the proposed action.
Effective Dates	A clear error in this element results in an overpayment or underpayment of benefits.
J) Are all payment dates correct?	Basic rules include 38 CFR 3.31, 3.114, 3.400-404 & 3.500-504.
Denials	
K1) Was all applicable evidence discussed?	Question K1 is self-explanatory.
K2) Was the basis of each decision explained?	Question K2 is self-explanatory.
NOTIFICATIONS	38 CFR 3.103 contains the basic rule. Claimants and their representatives are entitled to timely notice of any decision made by VA. This rule applies to both awards and disallowances.
L1) Was notification sent?	The appeal period does not begin until the claimant and representative are notified of the decision.
L2) Was the Power of Attorney indicated and correct?	The master record should be updated to include designation of the claimant's representative so that computer-generated notices are furnished to both.
L3) Was the notification correct?	Correspondence is VA's primary communication medium. Information must be complete and accurate.
L4) Were appeal rights included?	Notice of procedural and appellate rights are required following every decision. These may be furnished by attachment of VA Form 4107 or equivalent language in the body of the notification.

APPENDIX C

Attachments on the Department of Transportation's Balanced Scorecard

The following material was adapted from *Department of Transportation's Procurement Balanced Scorecard*, May 1999, www.dot.gov/ost/m60/scorecard/ppmsrev.htm.

FY00 DOT-WIDE PROCUREMENT PERFORMANCE MEASUREMENTS
(DOT's Balanced Scorecard)

Measurement	Pathway (Data Source)	Goal
Customer		
C1. % of Customer Satisfaction (weighted average of numbers C2–C4) **C2. Timeliness** **C3. Quality** **C4. Service Partnership**	Survey	85%
Employee		
E1. % of Employee Satisfaction (weighted average of nos. E2 and E3) **E2. % Satisfied with Work Environment** **E3. % Satisfied with Professionalism, Culture, Values, and Empowerment (Leadership/Management)**	Survey	80%
Internal Business Processes (IBPs)		
B1. Extent of Acquisition Excellence	Survey	TBD
B2. Extent of Mission Focus	Survey	TBD
B3. Ratio of Protests Sustained by GAO, COFC, and Other Dispute Resolution Venues	MIS (CICA Report, DOT Files)	TBD
B4. % of Actions Using Electronic Commerce	MIS (CIS, GSA/ECPO Report)	Increase by 5%

B5. % Achievement of Socio-economic Goals
      a. Small Businesses
      b. 8(a)s
      c. Small Disadvantaged Businesses
      d. Women-Owned Business Enterprises
	MIS (DOT Files, CIS)	TBD

B6. % Competitive Procurements of Total Procurements
  a. % competitive from all actions
  b. % competed actions from all available for compet.
	MIS (CIS)	TBD

B7. % of Purchase Card Transactions of Total Simplified Acquisition Actions	MIS (Bank Card Holder, SF 281)	87.5%
B8. Extent IBP Facilitates a Program That Effectively Applies and Complies with Statutory and Regulatory	Diagnostic, Executive Report	TBD
Learning and Growth		
L1. Extent of Reliable Management Information	Survey	TBD

L2. % Employees Meeting Mandatory Qualification Stds
  a. % meeting training requirements
  b. % meeting educational requirements
	MIS (Acquisition Career Develop. System)	Inc. by 50%
		Inc. by 5%

Finance		
F1. % Cost Benefit	Survey	TBD
F2. Amt of Cost Avoidance through Use of Purchase Cards	MIS (Bank Card Holder, SF 281)	TBD
F3. % of "Prompt Pay" Interest Paid versus Total $ Disbursed	MIS (DAFIS)	TBD
F4. % of Total Obligated $ Spent Purchasing Com. Items (CI)	MIS (CIS)	TBD
F5. % of Total $ Obligated for (CI) Buys from SB Concerns	MIS (CIS)	TBD
F6. Ratio of Cost to Spend	MIS (CIS), Exec. Report	TBD

Attachment B

SURVEY PATHWAY

INTRODUCTION

The Survey Pathway is the first path in DOT's Procurement Performance Management System. It is mainly a *qualitative* method for determining how we are progressing in meeting our goal of becoming a world class acquisition system. The Performance Measurement Assessment Tool (PMAT) is the foundation for the work under this Pathway and its concepts have been applied throughout DOTs BSC.

SURVEY PATHWAY METHODOLOGY

The measurement results in this path are based upon data derived from surveys. These surveys are developed by the Procurement Information Exchange (PIE) Council who have cognizance over this Pathway as chartered by the Procurement Management Council (PMC). When practicable, top-level measurements (e.g., customer and employee satisfaction) have a targeted goal against which the data results are compared.

Choosing Measurements. DOT uses three surveys—customer, employee, and manager self-assessment. The PIE Council, who reviews the surveys before their annual administration, determines DOT's "core questions." They, normally in conjunction with their PMC member, develop/select OA specific questions to be added to the surveys. However, only core question results are made a part of the BSC.

The measurement surveys are intended to be very different than conventional assessments. They have been structured for ease of use and minimal time for completion. The PIE Council members continually look for ways to increase the overall response rates by reducing the burden on the individuals responding to the surveys such as providing a fully automated survey process. The goal of the PIE Council is to ensure that only necessary questions are asked which will help to identify specific areas where the procurement process could improve. By reviewing the rating of the survey questions by the order of importance, the PIE Council is able to assess what areas are important to the customers and the employees. Care is taken to ensure that each survey is user-friendly to potentially increase the response rate. Also to maintain data integrity, the responses are completely anonymous.

Survey Rating. As noted above, the survey questions are weighted by order of importance as determined by the respondent. The responses are grouped to reflect the various perspectives of the BSC and a numeric rating is assigned to each based upon the level of customer, employee, or manager agreement. The benefit of this numeric rating is that the individual organizations can compare the changes over the years and set goals for future years.

The Senior Procurement Executive's office compiles the data and normally displays the results in graph or chart form for the operating administrations. It is the result of these surveys that can pinpoint areas needing attention and from which management direction for improved performance can flow.

Administering the Survey. The survey is administered through a Web-based application. The Office of the SPE has developed a BSC site that provides a unique entryway and location for the OA surveys. The SPE will meet with OA representatives annually to review the survey and develop a time-line for actions required to complete the surveys. The SPE will also provide information about techniques to improve response rates. The survey will be made available on the DOT/OA Website annually during November and December so that results can be collected and analyzed to support the GPRA reporting process.

CORE MEASUREMENTS

Attachment B1 reflects the quantifiable measurements and targeted goals (where stated) that will be used to gauge DOT's performance under the Survey Pathway. It is the scores of these core measurements that are incorporated within the BSC.

Attachment B1

SURVEY PATHWAY
(Core Measurements—Mainly Qualitative)

Measurement by Perspective	*DOT Goal (FY 00)*
CUSTOMER	
C1. % of Customer Satisfaction (weighted average of nos. C2–C4) **C2. Timeliness** **C3. Quality** **C4. Service Partnership**	85%

EMPLOYEE	
E1. % of Employee Satisfaction (weighted average of nos. E2 and E3) E2. Work Environment E3. Professionalism, Culture, Values, and Empowerment (Leadership/Management)	80%
INTERNAL BUSINESS PROCESSES	
B1. Acquisition Excellence B2. Extent of Mission Focus	TBD TBD
LEARNING AND GROWTH	
L1. Extent of Reliable Management Information	TBD
FINANCE	
F1. Cost Benefit	TBD

Attachment C

MANAGEMENT INFORMATION
SYSTEM (MIS) PATHWAY

INTRODUCTION

The MIS Pathway is the second path in DOT's Procurement Performance Management System. It is a *quantifiable* method for determining how we are progressing in meeting our goal of becoming a world class acquisition system.

MIS PATHWAY METHODOLOGY

The measurement results in this path are based upon data derived from management information systems normally developed and used within DOT such as the Contract Information System, the Financial Data System, and the Electronic Posting System. Each measurement has a targeted goal (when practicable) against which the data results are compared. This comparison indicates how well we are progressing toward our overall goal for a world class acquisition system.

Choosing Measurements. More than any other path, the measurements for this pathway relies [sic] heavily on the accuracy and availability of data systems. While this may limit our selection of measurements, it has not precluded the development of a balanced approach to viewing our progress. The measurements that we choose for this scorecard are encased within our targeted performance areas and may deal with special DOT interests, initiatives from outside organizations such as Congress, or issues of public policy. The specific measures are chosen by:

- **The Senior Procurement Executive (SPE).** These measurements are normally outgrowths from mandated issues from higher levels.
- **The Procurement Management Council in concert with the SPE.** These measurements involve areas of DOT wide interest and can help support budget requests for items of a common nature. This ONE DOT approach provides more leverage in budget negotiations.
- **Two or more Departments.** These measures may be derived through partnerships with other Departments for benchmarking purposes. To more effectively assess our progress, DOT participates in this type of endeavor.
- **Operating administrations.** Each OA can develop and implement their [sic] own measures based upon their [sic] unique needs.

Collecting MIS Data. Except for the "Cost to Spend" measure, collecting MIS data will normally be done annually in December and January and reflect the data results from the previous fiscal year. "Cost to Spend" will also be collected annually normally in November or December and utilize the "Executive Report" data collection tool.

CORE MEASUREMENTS

Attachment C1 reflects the quantifiable measurements and targeted goals (where stated) that will be used to gauge our performance under the MIS Pathway. The results of these core measurements will be integrated within the BSC.

Attachment C1

MANAGEMENT INFORMATION SYSTEM (MIS) PATHWAY
(Core Measurements—Quantifiable)

Measurements by Perspective (numbered and lettered in sequence with the Survey Pathway)	Data System	DOT Goal (FY 00)
INTERNAL BUSINESS PROCESSES		
B3. Ratio of Protests Sustained by GAO, COFC, and Other Dispute Resolution Venues	CICA Report, DOT Files	TBD
B4. % of Actions Using Electronic Commerce	CIS, GSA/ECPO Report	TBD

B5. % Achievement of Socio-economic Goals
  a. Small Businesses
  b. 8(a)s
  c. Small Disadvantaged Businesses Women-Owned Business Enterprises
	DOT Files, CIS	TBD

B6. % Competitive Procurements of Total Procurements	CIS	TBD
B7. % of Purchase Card Transactions of Total Simplified Acquisition Actions	Bank Card Holder & SF 281	87.5%
LEARNING AND GROWTH		

L2. % of Employees Meeting Mandatory Qualification Standards
  a. % meeting training requirements
  b. % meeting educational requirements
	Consolidated Personnel Management Information System	Increase by 50%
		Increase by 5%

FINANCE		
F2. Cost Avoidance through Use of Purchase Cards	Bank Card Holder & SF 281	TBD
F3. % of "Prompt Pay" Interest Paid versus Total Dollars Disbursed	DAFIS	TBD
F4. % of Total Obligated Dollars Spent Purchasing Commercial Items (CI)	CIS	TBD
F5. % of Total Dollars Obligated for CI Buys from Small Business Concerns	CIS	TBD
F6. Cost to Spend Ratio	CIS, Executive Report	TBD

DIAGNOSTIC PATHWAY
(Statutory and Regulatory Application and Compliance)

INTRODUCTION

It is the results of the third pathway in DOT's Procurement Performance Management System, the Diagnostic Pathway, that help us gauge how DOT contracting organizations are doing in applying and meeting applicable laws and regulations. This method permits each operating administration to choose the assessment approach to be used and the requirements to be evaluated.

DIAGNOSTIC METHODOLOGY

In the Diagnostic Pathway, one measurement is used—**Extent internal business processes facilitate a procurement program that effectively applies and complies with statute and regulation.** The results of this measurement can be determined by using one, both, or a combination of the assessment techniques below.

- **Process Assessment.** Within an organization's internal business processes there are many tools utilized to achieve a specific purpose. The Process Assessment examines the *adequacy of these tools*, whether electronic, hardcopy, or verbal, for institutionalizing and applying a process for compliance. It is these tools that, when used alone or in concert with others, help drive and sustain consistent and effective performance. The type of tools that may be examined include systems, procedures, policies, or processes, such as:

Knowledge Transfer	*Knowledge Tracking*
Training Program (e.g., classroom, on-the-job, refresher training)	Management Information Systems (e.g., Automated Procurement Systems)
Policy Letters and Memos (e.g., policy for receipt of procurement requests, document flow)	Procurement Measurement System (e.g., Percentage of Competitive Procurements)
Procedural Guidance or Manuals (e.g., Transportation Acquisition Manual)	Internal Monitoring Program (e.g., periodic self-assessments including random checks of procurement actions for actual compliance)
Electronic Commerce Systems (e.g., Contract Writing System, Electronic Posting System)	
Newsletters, Electronic Transmissions	
Delegations of Authority, Responsibility and Accountability	

- **Results Assessment.** This assessment indicates *if compliance is being achieved* throughout the contracting process. This assessment is accomplished by reviewing that information; whether electronic, hardcopy, or verbal, that verifies if the statutory and regulatory requirements *have been met*. Normally, this is done by reviewing the information (e.g., contract files) relevant to the procurement action. This assessment uses data collection devices such as requirements checklists (tailored to the assessment areas), sampling plan (defines information to be evaluated), electronic or manual data systems, and data spreadsheets (provides basis for any recommendation).

ASSESSMENT STEPS

When conducting a Process or Results Assessment, the following steps are recommended:

- *Determine which statutory and regulatory requirements are to be assessed.* A list of recommended assessment areas (which may be further refined) is provided in this section. It is important however, to keep abreast of any new laws or regulations that should be considered in the evaluation. While all requirements of law and regulation are not included in the list, many are contained within these broad areas. The assessment may include requirements targeted for OA improvement, of special interest to the administration, etc.
- *Determine which tools apply to the assessment.* This step aligns the tool with the specific statutory and/or regulatory requirement. For example, under the Process Assessment, an electronic writing system may be a tool used to assist *in applying* the proper provisions and clauses in a solicitation. For the Results Assessment, a checklist may be used to document if the proper provisions and clauses were *actually used* in a solicitation.
- *Determine which approach for assessment is to be used.* This step focuses on the many types of assessments that can be performed and the decision as to which is appropriate for the effort at hand. The various types of assessments include Internal Evaluations, OA Partnership Evaluations, etc. (see "Approaches for Assessment").
- *Develop an Assessment Plan.* The Plan may be developed in partnership with the evaluators and contains:
  - The statutory and regulatory requirements to be assessed.
  - The tools that will apply to each requirement and any instructions for obtaining/ accessing information for the evaluation (whether electronic, hardcopy, or verbal).
  - The approach to be used for the assessment and any guidelines including:
    - What and how much (sample population) is to be reviewed; and
    - How the evaluation results are to be presented (e.g., report, briefing).
  - Attachment D1 for completion by the evaluators (see "Rating Methodology").
- *Make available pertinent information to the evaluators.* Through management systems and other sources, the evaluators can determine what information (or individuals) needs to be accessed to accomplish the assessment and answer questions related to the application and compliance with law and regulation. This information may include hardcopy or electronic files or access to electronic systems.
- *Commence assessment and report results.* The assessment is conducted by the evaluation team and the results reported to the procurement manager. The evaluation, as a minimum, is to:
  - Validate if the internal business processes used facilitates a program that effectively applies and complies with statute and regulation;
  - Provide sufficient information (e.g., deficiencies found, recommended remedies) for a positive course of action for improving the agency's internal business processes; and
  - Provide a score for each statement on attachment D1 as it relates to the evaluation (see "Rating Methodology").

Executive Report. The data results given to the procurement manager are transferred (along with responses to the "Cost to Spend" (MIS Pathway) measure) to an electronic "Executive Report" submitted to the PMC members for completion or further distribution, as appropriate, in November or December of each year by the SPE's office.

RECOMMENDED ASSESSMENT AREAS

The following are recommended areas for evaluation:

- Using provisions and clauses (e.g., FAR and TAR) appropriately
  - Using funds as available and authorized
    - Integrating Acquisition Planning for an effective overall process
      - Using competitive procedures to the maximum extent
        - Using simplified acquisition procedures properly
          - Implementing socio-economic initiatives
            - Performing contract administration functions as required
              - Employing integrity in daily procurement operations

SCHEDULE FOR ASSESSMENTS

An assessment shall be conducted, as a minimum, every three years beginning in Fiscal Year (FY) 2000. *For OAs with many field offices, it is expected that this three-year interval will provide enough time for an assessment of a sufficient number of field offices for a reliable overall OA performance score.* If an evaluation indicates problems in specific areas, in subsequent years a partial evaluation targeting the problem area is recommended to determine if the strategic actions taken are resulting in improvement. For efficiency and consistency, the same evaluation team should conduct the partial evaluation. The rating methodology explained below will assist in gauging improvement progress.

APPROACHES FOR ASSESSMENT

There are various optional approaches to assess how the organization is performing. Most of the following evaluation approaches can be used singularly or in combination with another.

Self Evaluation

Internal Evaluation

OA Partnership Evaluation

Outside Independent Evaluation

Inspection Office Evaluation

Self Evaluation. This evaluation approach is conducted by the managers and/or contracting officials directly involved in the process or procurement action (e.g., solicitation development, contract award, contract administration) being assessed. This approach must be used in conjunction with another evaluation approach.

Internal Evaluation. This evaluation approach is conducted by personnel within the OA who can provide an objective examination of the process or actions to be reviewed. These personnel may be located within or outside the contracting office being assessed (e.g., DOT Headquarters office assessing their field offices).

OA Partnership Evaluation. This evaluation approach is accomplished by a partnering arrangement with another DOT OA, usually on a reciprocal basis. The review is to be objective; therefore, it is performed by personnel having no direct involvement with the process or actions being assessed. This type of evaluation can occur when one OA assesses another or when two or more OAs co-op their efforts in a team approach. An OA may also request the SPE's office to participate in an evaluation.

Outside Independent Evaluation. This evaluation approach is conducted by personnel outside DOT such as other Departments, independent organizations, and contractors. The evaluation is to be objective; therefore, it shall be performed by personnel having no direct involvement with the actions being evaluated.

Inspection Office Evaluation. This evaluation approach is conducted by offices chartered to inspect functional areas within an organization. They include the Inspector General and the General Accounting Office. This evaluation type applies when law and regulatory application and compliance issues are a substantial part of the evaluation.

RATING METHODOLOGY

The Diagnostic Pathway rating for the BSC is determined by using attachment D1.

Procurement Office score. The procurement office score is derived as follows:

- Evaluators respond to the statements in attachment D1 and record a team consensus score for each statement. The rating results are made a part of the deliverable at the end of each evaluation.
- The Procurement Management Council member or designee (e.g., senior procurement manager within the office evaluated) is to ensure the consensus scores *for each office assessed* in that year are transferred to the Executive's Report when it is administered in November or December. This needs to be recorded only in the year of an evaluation. The SPE's office will average the consensus scores for each assessed office to derive one overall measurement rating for that office.
- The evaluation team's rating is carried forward each year until another evaluation (including any partial evaluation) is done and new team ratings are posted.

OA score. The OA score is derived from the team consensus score. *For those OAs with field offices, the overall OA rating is calculated by averaging all office scores.* Therefore, an overall OA rating may change as the Headquarter and each additional field office is evaluated. To get a total OA score, it may take the full three-year cycle to evaluate all OA offices. *When the score is tallied each year for the BSC, the names of the offices comprising the OA score will be listed.*

DOT wide score. The DOT wide score is derived by averaging all OA scores and qualified to reflect the number of offices included in the score. Specific OA and field office names will not be published.

Attachment D1

DIAGNOSTIC PATHWAY
(Statutory and Regulatory Application and Compliance)

Measurements by Perspective
(numbered and lettered in sequence with the Survey and MIS Pathways)
B8. Extent Internal Business Processes Facilitate a Procurement Program That Effectively Applies and Complies with Statute and Regulation.

   a. The procurement office has implemented an effective internal monitoring process (e.g., self-assessment, quality action plan).

Strongly Agree	Agree	Disagree	Strongly Disagree
4	3	2	1

a. The procurement office provides adequate tools (e.g., on-the-job training, policy and procedural guidance, automated systems) to facilitate the effective application of and compliance with law and regulation.

Strongly Agree	Agree	Disagree	Strongly Disagree
4	3	2	1

a. The procurement office uses action plans and/or strategies for continuous improvement.

Strongly Agree	Agree	Disagree	Strongly Disagree
4	3	2	1

a. The evaluation covered sufficient statutory and regulatory requirements to reach a reliable conclusion as to the ability of the procurement office to effectively apply and comply with statute and regulation while supporting the organization's mission.

Strongly Agree	Agree	Disagree	Strongly Disagree
4	3	2	1

a. The evaluation covered a sufficient sampling of contract files, processes, systems, etc. to reach a reliable conclusion as to the ability of the procurement office to effectively apply and comply with statute and regulation while supporting the organization's mission.

Strongly Agree	Agree	Disagree	Strongly Disagree
4	3	2	1

NOTE: This scoresheet will be filled out by the evaluators for each office assessed and the results transferred by the PMC member or their [sic] designee as part of the Executive's Report requested in November or December.

Attachment E

TOOLS FOR ASSESSING PERFORMANCE

Some of the many tools available to gauge your improvement progress . . . include:

Benchmarking. Benchmarking, or comparing your performance against another, will provide an indication of how you are performing. It also serves as one input for developing target goals. However, as noted by the International Benchmarking Clearinghouse, the strength of benchmarking is not in identifying best performance, but in learning best practices. That is, it is important to identify, study, analyze, and adapt the successful practices that led to the performance. Understanding these successful practices helps you make better-informed decisions about where and how to change your organization. Also, by sharing what you have learned with others, enhances the opportunity for further Departmentwide improvement.

Tips for Benchmarking. Benchmarking can be performed with many groups including procurement offices: within your operating administration (OA), outside your OA (i.e., other OAs), within other Departments, or within different industry groups. DOT will be periodically benchmarking with other Departments on a Departmentwide basis. To make valid comparisons, you need to consider how the others being benchmarked are similar and different. Common factors to consider include:

- Is the total size and budget similar?
- Is the amount spent on acquisition comparable?
- Is the percent of total budget spent on acquisition similar?
- Does the other have a similar mission or work of comparable complexity?
- Are the products and services acquired similar?

The Business Case. In addition to strategic feedback and learning, you can also use the BSC to build a strong, sound business case to support proposals for changes or requests for resources. The BSC can illuminate links between strategies, measures, and expected outcomes at different levels in the organization, and across different operational components. This provides a framework for explaining how and why a proposed change will benefit the organization and the expected effect on linked components. For example, an operating administration or the Department in a "ONE DOT" approach, can use the BSC to support budget requests by demonstrating how funding would improve Departmentwide efficiency and also benefit program mission accomplishment.

Public Policy and Compliance. BSC information can be used to evaluate the level of compliance with law, regulation, and public policy initiatives. DOT uses the BSC to achieve this purpose. When BSC measures are properly aligned with your objectives, review efforts should be focused where they will have the most benefit. Reviews should analyze the cause of concern and identify appropriate remedies (e.g., recommending changes in operational practices, clarifying existing or developing new policies, or eliminating or revising policies that create problems or activities that are non-value-added). The BSC also provides a framework for reporting to the agency head, Congress, or other higher level offices.

Self-diagnosis. You can use the results for "self-diagnosis." BSC data together with other reports and statistics can help you anticipate and resolve issues before they become problems, or at least minimize the effect of problems by early action. Information from other reports and statistics may also indicate the need to adjust BSC strategies and measures.

Cross-functional Problem Solving. By illuminating the links between strategies, measures, and expected outcomes at different levels, and across different operational components, the BSC can encourage cross-functional problem solving. For example, you may identify a policy that impedes your ability to accomplish a certain objective. You could raise the issue with the cognizant office, using the BSC to demonstrate the cause-and-effect relationship, and work together with the appropriate management to produce a solution. Another example is within an acquisition office—you may work with finance to establish an electronic system for receiving and processing invoices which benefits the performance of both organizations.

Enhancing Strategic Feedback and Learning for Future Results. A necessary ingredient for continuous improvement is discussing how past results were achieved and whether their expectations for the future remain on track. Changes in the environment (e.g., new technology, legislative initiatives) may create new opportunities or risks not anticipated when your initial strategies were developed. If you followed established strategies, but did not achieve target results, you should examine internal capabilities and assess whether the underlying strategies remain valid. Based on such analyses, you may adjust or redirect your strategies or identify new ones. This focus serves as a foundation for effective process improvement and risk management. It also completes a feedback loop that supports decision-making at all levels of the organization.

Gap Management. Gaps between your strategic objectives/goals and actual achievement can be detected by using performance results. The root causes of these gaps can be analyzed and corrective action developed and implemented. Whenever there is a gap between current results and your objectives, it is an opportunity for process improvement. This may require reengineering and/or redesigning of your process. Analyzing how a process flows is especially useful when BSC results indicate performance gaps in the areas of timeliness, costs, or efficiency. Understanding which key processes need the most attention, and then aggressively addressing the differences between current performance and the desired end state, is a hallmark of successful organizations.

Risk Management. The BSC can be used as a risk management tool where it creates an infrastructure within which key managers are held accountable for results. DOT uses the BSC for this purpose. This is done by shifting the emphasis to a risk-based approach that diagnoses systemic problems, evaluates effectiveness, and links performance to consequences in order to strike a proper balance between risk and return. In other words, risk management (and the BSC) is more strategic than reactive.

OA and Departmentwide Improvements. Establishing organizational improvement structures and procedures may help implement performance improvements, and to make a genuine commitment to performance management. After the BSC results have been analyzed, you may wish to consider forming teams for the areas you have targeted for improvement (e.g., "Timeliness," as addressed in the customer survey). The team should consist of major stakeholders to ensure that all participants in the acquisition process become involved in (and reach consensus on) system improvements. Depending on the performance issue, the team might consist of acquisition employees alone, acquisition employees and customers (cross-functional), or acquisition employees and managers.

REFERENCES AND RESOURCES

The following were utilized as a resource in writing this document:

Benchmarking: Leveraging "Best Practice Strategies." International Benchmarking Clearinghouse, A White Paper for Senior Management, based on the internationally acclaimed 1995 study: Organizing & Managing Benchmarking.

Keeping Score, Mark Graham Brown, Quality Resources, 1996.

Procurement Executives' Association, Guide to a Balanced Scorecard Performance Management Methodology, PEA chartered interagency team, 1998.

Quality in Contracting: "QUIC" Guidebook, Integrated Acquisition Performance Measurement Program, U.S. Department of the Interior, October 1996.

Quality Management Implementation Guidelines, U.S. Department of Energy, July 1997

Serving the American Public: Best Practices in Performance Measurement. Benchmarking Study Report, National Performance Review, June 1997.

The Balanced Scorecard: Translating Strategy into Action. Robert S. Kaplan and David P. Norton, Harvard Business School Press, 1996.

Using the Balanced Scorecard as a Strategic Management System. Robert S. Kaplan and David P. Norton, *Harvard Business Review,* January-February 1996.

APPPENDIX D

Balanced Scorecard for a Contractor

The information presented in this appendix is adapted from a November 4, 1998 briefing by John Hirsch and Joseph Montgomery of the Strategic Effectiveness Group, LLC (see Chapter 14). It is presented with the approval of Mr. Hirsch.

SECTION TWO APPLYING THE MODEL: CREATING A BALANCED SCORECARD FOR A HYPOTHETICAL HANFORD CONTRACTOR

Preliminary Steps in Balanced Scorecard Preparation

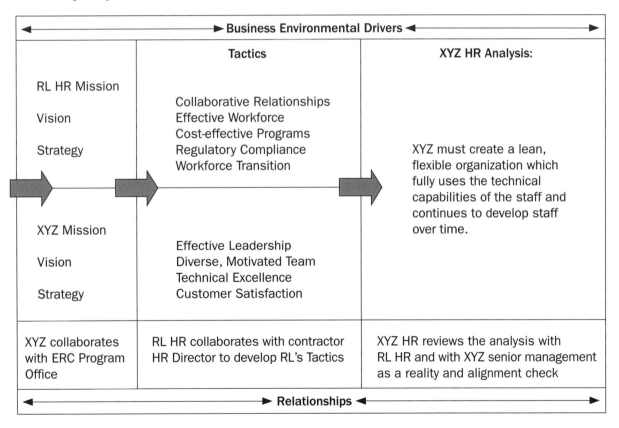

Understanding RL HR and Contractor HR Drivers

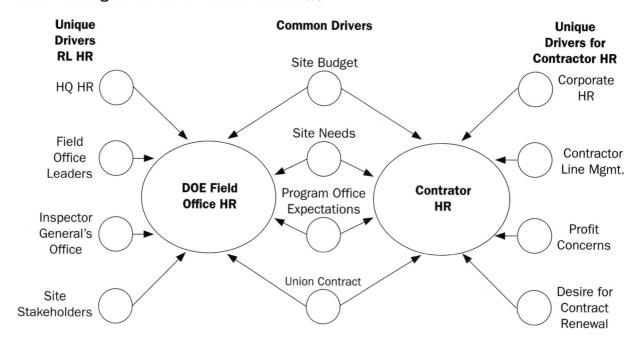

Using Desired Organizational Characteristics To Drive Assessment, Goals, Tactics, and Measures

Org. Characteristics	How Do We Compare w/ Best practices?	Performance Targets	HR Actions	Measures
Empowered Teams Productive workforce Strong culture, values Low overheads				
XYZ HR and RL HR collaborate on desired characteristics	XYZ HR and RL HR collaborate, reach consensus	Collaborate, reach consensus	XYZ decides which actions it wishes to take	Consensus on the measures, incentives

◄─────────────────► Relationships ◄──────────────►

Possible Missions for Contractors

- Environmental restoration/cleanup
- Research and development
- Defense production
- Each mission will require its own distinct vision of success, strategy, and tactics

(XYZ mission is environmental restoration and cleanup)

Aligning XYZ Mission, Vision, Strategy

	XYZ	**RL–HR**
Mission	**Assess and clean up hazardous contamination**	**As a public steward, oversee contractors to provide the workforce needed for effective, efficient cleanup**
Vision	**Highly efficient, effective, technically advanced, partnering, leadership, teamwork**	**Collaborative relations w/all parties; capable, cost-effective workforce, compliance w/regs. and goals of workforce transition**
Strategy	**High tech. with strong customer linkages, project mgmt. skills**	**Tightly linked w/customers & suppliers (contractors)**

Primary Tactics to Support Strategy

XYZ Tactics for Innovation Strategy
　　Developing Effective Leadership
　　Creating a Diverse, Motivated Team
　　Ensuring Technical Excellence
　　Building Customer Satisfaction

RL-HR Tactics for Tight Linkages Strategy
　　Creating Collaborative Relationships
　　Promoting an Effective Workforce
　　Promoting Cost Effective Programs
　　Requiring Regulatory Compliance
　　Requiring Workforce Transition

Aligning XYZ Mission, Vision, Strategy

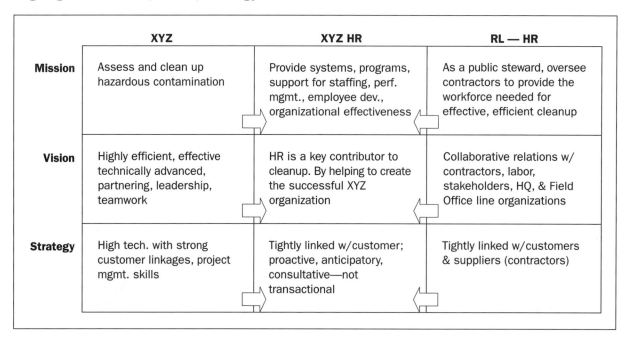

	XYZ	XYZ HR	RL — HR
Mission	Assess and clean up hazardous contamination	Provide systems, programs, support for staffing, perf. mgmt., employee dev., organizational effectiveness	As a public steward, oversee contractors to provide the workforce needed for effective, efficient cleanup
Vision	Highly efficient, effective technically advanced, partnering, leadership, teamwork	HR is a key contributor to cleanup. By helping to create the successful XYZ organization	Collaborative relations w/ contractors, labor, stakeholders, HQ, & Field Office line organizations
Strategy	High tech. with strong customer linkages, project mgmt. skills	Tightly linked w/customer; proactive, anticipatory, consultative—not transactional	Tightly linked w/customers & suppliers (contractors)

XYZ Organizational Characteristics Desired for Success of Mission

1. Decentralized, highly flexible empowered project teams that share skills and functional support via a matrix structure
2. Workforce which is very productive and has right KSAs
3. A culture which focuses on:
   - Performance guided by strong values: safety, integrity, innovation, and quality
   - Employee development: know-how for good performance on current job, planning for next job
   - Rewards & recognition for performance/results
   - Regular measurement of performance
4. Low overheads: low ratio of support to productive labor and lower costs of staff

Desired Organizational Characteristics Drive HR Assessment, Goals, Tactics, and Measures— Example

Organizational Characteristic	How Do We Compare to Best Practices Applicable to This Site?	Perf. Targets	HR Actions	Perf. Measures	BSC Quadrant
Empowered Flexible Teams	· Highly effective, but need to improve sharing staff expertise across projects · Some self-managed teams (SMTs)	· Maintain effectiveness but 10% greater sharing · 10% more SMTs	· Establish baseline · Create tracking mechanism · Develop reports to recognize sharing managers	· Survey of project mgr. perceptions; · % staff on >1 project · # SMTs	Work processes
Low Overhead	Generally favorable, except 15% above market comparator for all benefit costs	Reduce benefit costs by 10% next year	· Increase insurance deductibles · Increase stop-loss · Study other benefit programs for later actions	Deductible % Increase · # programs evaluated · Benefits expense factor	Finance
Effective Reward and Recognition Program	· Current programs are ad hoc, lack formalization · R&R programs need to be strategically tied to achieving the mission, reinforcing the business strategy, producing the desired results	· Formalized programs in place · Direct links w/strategy, desired outcomes, & culture	· Form line/HR employee team to design program · Obtain Gvt/DOE approval · Obtain union support as necessary · Implement program · Communicate to staff	· % time over schedule · Survey—mgmt, staff perceptions · $ value of awards (per capita) · # staff recognized (% of total)	Culture
A workforce that has the right KSAs for current jobs and is building skills for transition to the next job	· Workforce has right skills for today, but inadequate attention to the next job · Need meaningful, individualized development plans for exempt staff with most resources to high-potentials · Need planned skill enhancement programs related to new technologies for hourly staff	· Effective planning for next job · Mentoring for high potentials · Skill progs. in place	· Create a tailored, all staff dev. program · Obtain sr mgt approval · Pilot train hi-pots to create plan · Establish union/mgt team to develop skills program · Pilot with one skill	· % of hi-pots with dev. plans · Line mgt. sat. with dev. process · Pilot group sat. with perceived enhancement of skills	Culture

Organizational Characteristic	How Do We Compare to Best Practices Applicable to This Site?	Perf. Targets	HR Actions	Perf. Measures	BSC Quadrant
Support functions aligned with line organizations	Some alignment, especially in election/recruiting; HR tends to take on "policeman" role with line to get compliance with rules, rather than true service orientation. Tendency for adversarial relationships to result.	Line perceives step-function improvement in support orientation of "X" %	• Assess support orientation of each HR service area • Create a plan for achieving alignment in main functions • Assign accountable staff to each project • Solicit line input • Solicit line fdbk on progress	Survey—line perceptions of support for their needs; progress perceived	Culture

Sort Measures into a Draft BSC

Work Processes	**Culture**
• Project manager perceptions of sharing technical expertise* • # staff on >1 project	• % time over schedule for R&R • Survey—staff perceptions of R&R, development process* • $ value of awards, # recognition • # hi-pots with plans • Pilot group satisfaction
Customer Satisfaction	**Financial Goals**
• HR role effectiveness:* survey—executives; managers; employees; DOE-RL	• Increase in deductibles • # benefits programs evaluated • Benefits expense factor* • Budget for improvement projects • Revenue/FTE; expenses/FTE
*Indicates measures incentivized by DOE	

Summary

- Contractor HR organizations will be asked to create an HR BSC
- The BSC requires a logical, step-by-step development process that focuses on how HR supports organizational needs
- There are several decisions to be made, including desired level of performance compared with Best Practices
- The BSC development process provides major benefits to the HR function

Index

A

accountability, 145, 226
acquisition excellence, 253
American Society for Public
    Administration, 223

B

Balanced Scorecard (BSC)
    customer perspective, 6–7
    financial perspective, 5–6
    history, 2
    internal business
        perspective, 7–8
    learning and growth
        perspective, 8–10
balancing measures, best
    practices, 148–149
benchmarking, 262–263
best practices
    accountability, 145
    balancing measures, 148–
      149
    connect the dots, 145
    data, 145
    leadership role, 145
    lessons learned, 147
    measures, results-oriented,
      144
    overview, 143–144
    perspectives, 149–151
    purpose of studying, 146
BSC. *See* Balanced Scorecard
budget misalignment, 227
business case, 263

C

cause and effect, 230
clientele requirements, 264
Clinger-Cohen Act, 153
collaborative relationships,
    227
Commercial Off-the-Shelf
    (COTS) products, 12
competency, workforce, 225
competitive procurement,
    254
congruence, multiple
    programs, 224
connect the dots, best
    practices, 145
consistency, lack of, 230
contractors
    mission, 268–270
    organizational
      characteristics, 271–272
    preparation, 267
core competencies, 227
cost avoidance, 253, 257
COTS. *See* Commercial Off-
    the-Shelf products
customer loyalty, 61–62, 70
customer perspective, 6–7
customer satisfaction,
    48–49, 253, 255

D

data, best practices, 145
decision makers, 230

Department of Energy (DOE)
    balanced scorecard,
      overview, 219–222
    human resource planning,
      213–214
    measurement perspective,
      232
    preparation, 216–218
    requirements, 214–215
Department of
    Transportation (DOT)
    acquisition, 197–201
    Diagnostic Pathway, 258–
      262
    Management Information
      System (MIS) Pathway,
      256–257
    measurement perspective,
      232
    performance
      management, 201–203
    planning model, 196
    policy principles, 192–195
    procurement balanced
      scorecard, 191–192
    procurement performance
      measures, 253–254
    strategic path, 195–196
    Survey Pathway, 254–256
    tools, performance
      assessment, 262–264
dispute resolution, 85–86
DOE. *See* Department of
    Energy
DOT. *See* Department of
    Transportation
drivers, 225

E

electronic commerce, 253
employee potential, 49,
    62–63, 70
employee satisfaction, 253,
    256
environmental assessment,
    14–15, 18, 31

F

Federal Aviation
    Administration Logistic
    Center (FAALC)
    1994 Strategic Plan
        overview, 11
    1997 Strategic Plan
        overview, 16
    1999-2000 Strategic Plan
        overview, 26
    action plan, 15
    business model, 15
    current business model,
        233–234
    customer perspective, 24,
        35
    customers, 237
    environmental
        assessment, 14–15, 18,
        31
    financial stakeholder
        perspective, 24, 36
    future business model,
        234–235
    gap analysis, 15, 235
    implementation, 15
    internal business
        perspective, 25, 37
    learning and innovation
        perspective, 25, 38
    lines of business, 237
    logistics, 236
    measurement perspective,
        231
    mission, 19, 28–29, 237
    organizational values, 20,
        30

process, 27, 29
    strategy development, 15,
        21, 32–34, 235–236
    vision, 28
financial perspective, 5–6
financial stakeholder
    perspective, 24, 36

G

GAO. *See* General
    Accounting Office
gap analysis, 15, 235
gap management, 264
General Accounting Office
    (GAO), 1
    customer needs, 169–172
    data collection and
        analysis, 163
    decision making, 163
    goals, 164–166
    innovation and learning,
        172–173
    IT Performance
        Management, 161–162
    measurement perspective,
        132
    objectives and measures,
        166–167
    practice areas, 162–167
    results chain, 162
    strategic needs, 167–169
General Services
    Administration (GSA),
    153–159, 232
Global Positioning Satellite
    (GPS), 12
goals, stakeholders, 264
Government Performance
    and Results Act of 1993
    (GPRA), 1, 79
GPRA. *See* Government
    Performance and Results
    Act of 1993
GPS. *See* Global Positioning
    Satellite
GSA. *See* General Services
    Administration

H

human resource planning,
    213–214

I

ICAD. *See* Integrated
    Computer Assisted
    Detection
Immigration and
    Naturalization Service
    (INS), 157
Information Technology,
    General Services
    Administration
    Clinger-Cohen Act, 153
    goals and objectives,
        linking to, 154–157
    Integrated Computer
        Assisted Detection, 157–
        158
innovation, 50, 66, 70
INS. *See* Immigration and
    Naturalization Service
Integrated Computer
    Assisted Detection (ICAD),
    157–158
Interagency Working Group
    on Performance
    Management
    Establish Accountability,
        131–133, 135–136, 140
    Expect Excellence, 129–
        131, 135–140
    overview, 127–129
    Take Timely Action, 133–
        134, 136, 140–142
internal business
    perspective, 7–8, 25, 37
internal business processes,
    253, 257
Internal Revenue Service
    (IRS)
    Automated Clearing
        House (ACH), 89
    Balanced Measurement
        System, 90–107

Commissioner's testimony, 87–90
course of action, 101–102
Customer Service Task Force, 89
diagnostic tools, 93–95
E-FILE campaign, 89
Electronic Returns Originators (ERO), 89
Executive Management Support System, 100
goals, 96–98
management model, 92–93
measurement perspective, 231
modernization, 88–89
Organizational Performance Management, 107–113
performance evaluation, 98–100
plan development, 95–96
problem definition, 101
small businesses, 90
telephone service, 90
IRS. *See* Internal Revenue Service

K

key practices
accountability, 229
American Society for Public Administration, 223
cause and effect, 228
challenges, 230
clientele responsibilities, 224
Coast Guard example, 227
drivers and results, 225
logic model, 228
means and strategies, 226
mission and goals, 226
overview, 223–224
performance-based management, 227
program delivery partners, 229
public governance responsibilities, 224
results, delivering, 228

L

leadership role, best practices, 145
learning and growth perspective, 8–10
local reviews, 83–84
logistics, 236

M

management information, 254
measurement perspectives, 231–232
measures, results-oriented, 144
mission focus, 253
mission statements, 226

N

National Airspace System, 12
National Highway Traffic Safety Administration, 228
National Oceanic and Atmospheric Administration (NOAA)
acquisitions, 207–208
customers, 206, 208–209
human resources, 209–212
inputs and outputs, 206, 208–209
measurement perspective, 232
measures of output, 210
perspectives, 206, 208–209
suppliers, 206, 208–209
systems, 205–206
National Partnership for Reinventing Government, 143
national reviews, 83
Naval Undersea Warfare Center (NUWC)
1998 Strategic Plan, 41–52
balanced performance measures, 44, 67–68
charter, 46
customer loyalty, 61–62, 70
customer satisfaction, 48–49
employee potential, 49, 62–63, 70
improvements, 63–64, 70
innovation, 50, 66, 70
management process, 51–52
measurement perspective, 231
mission, 46, 58, 70
Newport Division 1998 Strategic Plan, 53–68
Newport Division 1998 Strategic Plan Brochure, 69–71
Newport Division 5-Year Planning Process, 72–77
operating principles, 47–48, 59–60
ownership costs, lowering, 50
products, 65–66, 70
responsiveness, 49
Senior Management Team, 43
strategic goals, 44–45, 57–58
Undersea Warfare, 43
vision, 46, 70
Navy Program Executive Office for Information Technology (PEO/IT)
ITC Performance Blueprint, 123–126

ITC Strategic Direction,
    120–122
SEO/MP, 115–119
Non-developmental Items
    (NDI), 12
NUWC. *See* Naval Undersea
    Warfare Center

O

ownership costs, lowering, 50

P

P&L. *See* profit and loss
    statements
PEA. *See* Procurement
    Executives' Association
PEO/IT. *See* Navy Program
    Executive Office for
    Information Technology
performance plans,
    requirements for, 1
perspectives, best practices,
    149–151
PIE. *See* Procurement
    Information Exchange
Principle of Guardianship
    Files (PGF), 81
problem solving, cross-
    functional, 263
processes, day to day, 226
procurement balanced
    scorecard, 191–192
Procurement Executives'
    Association (PEA)
    data collection, 188–191
    experience, 184
    goals, 182–184
    implementation, 178–179
    methodology, 176–177
    mission, 182
    performance
        management, 175–176
    performance measures,
        181
    perspectives, 177–178
    strategy, 182

success, achieving, 179–181
    vision, 182
Procurement Information
    Exchange (PIE), 254
profit and loss (P&L)
    statements, 2
public governance
    responsibilities, 224
public policy, 263

R

responsiveness, 49
results chain, 162
results, delivering, 228
risk management, 264

S

self-diagnosis, 263
Senior Executive Service
    (SES), 3, 231
Senior Procurement
    Executive (SPE), 256
SEO/IMP. *See* Systems
    Executive Office for
    Manpower and Personnel
service partnership, 253, 255
SES. *See* Senior Executive
    Service
small businesses, 253, 257
small disadvantaged
    businesses, 253, 257
socio-economic goals, 253
SPE. *See* Senior Procurement
    Executive
stakeholders, 224
STAR. *See* Systematic
    Technical Accuracy
    Review process, VBA
stove pipes, 225
strategic plans, requirements
    for, 1
supplier management, 265
support responsibilities, 224
Systematic Technical
    Accuracy Review (STAR)
    process, VBA

analysis, review results,
    84–85
assessment, local review
    process, 85
compensation and
    pension claims, 79–80
core authorization, 81
core ratings, 80–81
dispute resolution, 85–86
errors, 82–83
local reviews, 83–84
national reviews, 83
Principle of Guardianship
    Files (PGF), 81
procedures, 81–82
Systems Executive Office for
    Manpower and Personnel
    (SEO/MP), 115–119, 231

T

timeliness, 253, 255
tools, performance
    assessment, 262–264

U

Undersea Warfare, 43

V

Veterans Benefits
    Administration (VBA)
    STAR authorization
        checklist, 246–252
    STAR rating checklist,
        239–245
    Systematic Technical
        Accuracy Review (STAR)
        process, 79–86

W

women-owned business
    enterprises, 253, 257
work environment, 256
workforce, competency, 225